Integrating Firearm Injury Prevention into Health Care

Proceedings of a Joint Workshop of the National Academies of Sciences, Engineering, and Medicine; Northwell Health; and PEACE Initiative

Joe Alper, Rose Marie Martinez, and Dara Rosenberg, *Rapporteurs*

Board on Population Health and Public Health Practice

Health and Medicine Division

Proceedings of a Workshop

THE NATIONAL ACADEMIES PRESS 500 Fifth Street, NW Washington, DC 20001

This activity was supported by Northwell Health and the PEACE Initiative. Any opinions, findings, conclusions, or recommendations expressed in this publication do not necessarily reflect the views of any organization or agency that provided support for the project.

International Standard Book Number-13: 978-0-309-69349-3
International Standard Book Number-10: 0-309-69349-7
Digital Object Identifier: https://doi.org/10.17226/26707

This publication is available from the National Academies Press, 500 Fifth Street, NW, Keck 360, Washington, DC 20001; (800) 624-6242 or (202) 334-3313; http://www.nap.edu.

Copyright 2022 by the National Academy of Sciences. National Academies of Sciences, Engineering, and Medicine and National Academies Press and the graphical logos for each are all trademarks of the National Academy of Sciences. All rights reserved.

Printed in the United States of America.

Suggested citation: National Academies of Sciences, Engineering, and Medicine. 2022. *Integrating firearm injury prevention into health care: Proceedings of a joint workshop of the National Academies of Sciences, Engineering, and Medicine; Northwell Health; and PEACE Initiative*. Washington, DC: The National Academies Press. https://doi.org/10.17226/26707.

The **National Academy of Sciences** was established in 1863 by an Act of Congress, signed by President Lincoln, as a private, nongovernmental institution to advise the nation on issues related to science and technology. Members are elected by their peers for outstanding contributions to research. Dr. Marcia McNutt is president.

The **National Academy of Engineering** was established in 1964 under the charter of the National Academy of Sciences to bring the practices of engineering to advising the nation. Members are elected by their peers for extraordinary contributions to engineering. Dr. John L. Anderson is president.

The **National Academy of Medicine** (formerly the Institute of Medicine) was established in 1970 under the charter of the National Academy of Sciences to advise the nation on medical and health issues. Members are elected by their peers for distinguished contributions to medicine and health. Dr. Victor J. Dzau is president.

The three Academies work together as the **National Academies of Sciences, Engineering, and Medicine** to provide independent, objective analysis and advice to the nation and conduct other activities to solve complex problems and inform public policy decisions. The National Academies also encourage education and research, recognize outstanding contributions to knowledge, and increase public understanding in matters of science, engineering, and medicine.

Learn more about the National Academies of Sciences, Engineering, and Medicine at **www.nationalacademies.org**.

Consensus Study Reports published by the National Academies of Sciences, Engineering, and Medicine document the evidence-based consensus on the study's statement of task by an authoring committee of experts. Reports typically include findings, conclusions, and recommendations based on information gathered by the committee and the committee's deliberations. Each report has been subjected to a rigorous and independent peer-review process and it represents the position of the National Academies on the statement of task.

Proceedings published by the National Academies of Sciences, Engineering, and Medicine chronicle the presentations and discussions at a workshop, symposium, or other event convened by the National Academies. The statements and opinions contained in proceedings are those of the participants and are not endorsed by other participants, the planning committee, or the National Academies.

Rapid Expert Consultations published by the National Academies of Sciences, Engineering, and Medicine are authored by subject-matter experts on narrowly focused topics that can be supported by a body of evidence. The discussions contained in rapid expert consultations are considered those of the authors and do not contain policy recommendations. Rapid expert consultations are reviewed by the institution before release.

For information about other products and activities of the National Academies, please visit www.nationalacademies.org/about/whatwedo.

PLANNING COMMITTEE FOR THE WORKSHOP ON FACILITATING THE INTEGRATION OF FIREARM INJURY PREVENTION INTO HEALTH CARE[1]

ANDRE CAMPBELL, Professor of Surgery; Vice Chair for Diversity, Equity, and Inclusion; and Director, University of California, San Francisco Surgical Critical Care Fellowship; University of California, San Francisco School of Medicine; Attending Trauma Surgeon, Zuckerberg San Francisco General Hospital and Trauma Center

ERICA FORD, Founder and Chief Executive Officer, LIFE Camp, Inc.

KAYLA A. HICKS, Chief Executive Officer, Sustain Equity Group

KYLEANNE HUNTER, Assistant Professor of Military and Strategic Studies, Strategy and Welfare Center, U.S. Air Force Academy; RAND Corporation

SANDEEP KAPOOR, Assistant Vice President, Addiction Services and Director of Screening, Brief Intervention, and Referral to Treatment, Northwell Health; Assistant Professor of Medicine, Donald and Barbara Zucker School of Medicine at Hofstra/Northwell

PETER MASIAKOS, Director, Pediatric Trauma Services and Codirector, Center for Gun Violence Prevention, Massachusetts General Hospital; Associate Professor of Surgery, Harvard Medical School

MEGAN RANNEY, Academic Dean, School of Public Health, Brown University; Director of the Brown-Lifespan Center for Digital Health; Professor of Behavioral and Social Sciences and Endowed Professor of Emergency Medicine, Warren Alpert Medical School of Brown University

JOSEPH SAKRAN, Director of Emergency General Surgery, Vice Chair for Clinical Operations, and Associate Professor of Surgery and Nursing, Johns Hopkins University

CHETHAN SATHYA, Director, Center for Gun Violence Prevention, Northwell Health; Associate Medical Director of Trauma and Surgical Director of Pediatric Critical Care, Cohen Children's Medical Center; Assistant Professor of Surgery, Donald and Barbara Zucker School of Medicine at Hofstra/Northwell

---

[1] The National Academies of Sciences, Engineering, and Medicine's planning committees are solely responsible for organizing the workshop, identifying topics, and choosing speakers. The responsibility for the published Proceedings of a Workshop rests with the workshop rapporteurs and the institution.

Project Staff

ROSE MARIE MARTINEZ, Senior Board Director on Population Health and Public Health Practice, and Director, Roundtable on Health Literacy
GRACE READING, Senior Program Assistant
DARA ROSENBERG, Research Associate
Y. CRYSTI PARK, Program Coordinator

Consultant

JOE ALPER, Consulting Writer

Reviewers

This Proceedings of a Workshop was reviewed in draft form by individuals chosen for their diverse perspectives and technical expertise. The purpose of this independent review is to provide candid and critical comments that will assist the National Academies of Sciences, Engineering, and Medicine in making each published proceedings as sound as possible and to ensure that it meets the institutional standards for quality, objectivity, evidence, and responsiveness to the charge. The review comments and draft manuscript remain confidential to protect the integrity of the process.

We thank the following individuals for their review of this proceedings:

STEPHEN W. HARGARTEN, Medical College of Wisconsin
JULIE PARSONNET, Stanford University

Although the reviewers listed above provided many constructive comments and suggestions, they were not asked to endorse the content of the proceedings nor did they see the final draft before its release. The review of this proceedings was overseen by **BOBBIE BERKOWITZ,** University School of Nursing, University of Washington. She was responsible for making certain that an independent examination of this proceedings was carried out in accordance with standards of the National Academies and that all review comments were carefully considered. Responsibility for the final content rests entirely with the rapporteurs and the National Academies. We also thank staff member **MEREDITH YOUNG,** Associate Program Officer, for reading and providing helpful comments on this manuscript.

Acknowledgments

The National Academies of Sciences, Engineering, and Medicine's Board on Population Health and Public Health Practice wishes to express its sincere gratitude to the members of the planning committee, who collaborated to ensure a workshop complete with informative presentations and rich discussions. The planning committee also thanks the speakers and moderators, who generously shared their expertise and their time with workshop participants. Finally, a special thanks to staff members Grace Reading and Crysti Park for their support of workshop activities.

Contents

BOX, FIGURES, AND TABLE   xiii

ACRONYMS AND ABBREVIATIONS   xv

1   INTRODUCTION   1
    Statement of Task, 2
    Opening Remarks, 3
    Organization of the Workshop, 6

2   FRAMING THE ISSUE: FIREARM INJURIES AND
    HEALTH CARE'S ROLE IN DEPOLARIZING A PUBLIC
    HEALTH CRISIS   9

3   HEALTH CARE STRATEGIES TO REDUCE FIREARM
    INJURY AND MORTALITY   15
    Investigating the Pipeline Through Community Partnerships,
        Intentionality, and Collaboration, 15
    The American College of Surgeons Committee on Trauma's
        ISAVE Initiative, 19
    The BulletPoints Project, 25
    Discussion, 28

4 BARRIERS AND FACILITATORS TO IMPLEMENTING
HOSPITAL-BASED FIREARM INJURY PREVENTION
STRATEGIES IN URBAN AND RURAL COMMUNITIES 31
Implementing Firearm Safety Promotion Programs in Pediatric
  Primary Care, 31
Hospital and Community Violence Intervention Propagation in
  the South: Unique Needs, Considerations, and Challenges, 34
Temple University Hospital's Cradle to Grave Program, 39
Acclivus Violence Prevention Services, 41
Discussion, 43

5 COLLABORATING WITH COMMUNITIES TO IMPROVE
HEALTH CARE SYSTEM IMPLEMENTATION SUCCESS
AND DESTIGMATIZE GUN VIOLENCE PREVENTION 45
The Bullet Related Injury Clinic, 45
Walk the Talk America: At the Intersection of Guns and Mental
  Health, 46
LIVE FREE USA, 47
Discussion, 49

6 DEFINING A FIREARMS VIOLENCE PREVENTION
ROAD MAP FOR HOSPITAL AND HEALTH SYSTEMS 53
How the Panelists Became Involved in Firearm Injury
  Prevention, 53
Successes and Challenges, 57
Thinking About Evaluation, 59
Transforming Communities to Prevent Firearm Violence, 60

7 CLOSING COMMENTS 63

APPENDIXES

A REFERENCES 67
B WORKSHOP AGENDA 73
C STATEMENT OF TASK 79
D BIOGRAPHICAL SKETCHES OF THE SPEAKERS AND
  MODERATORS 81

Box, Figures, and Table

BOX

6-1 Firearms Violence Prevention Road Map Highlights, 54

FIGURES

3-1 Federal Housing Authority's practice of redlining denied mortgages to Black and low-income populations, 16
3-2 Federal Housing Authority mortgage lending map of Los Angeles County showing redlined areas, 20
3-3 Social determinants of health, 21
3-4 Maps of Los Angeles County showing environmental health risk, homicides, unemployment rate, diabetic amputations, poverty level, and grocery store locations/food deserts by neighborhood, 22

4-1 The implementation science subway, 32
4-2 Firearm homicide rates by state per 100,000, 2020, 35
4-3 Area Deprivation Index for South Carolina, with red areas being the most disadvantaged regions and blue the least disadvantaged, 36

TABLE

3-1 Individuals Seen for Gunshot Wounds or Stabbing by Hospital in Boston, 17

Acronyms and Abbreviations

BMC	Boston Medical Center
BRIC	Bullet Related Injury Clinic
CDC	Centers for Disease Control and Prevention
HAVI	Health Alliance for Violence Intervention
HIPAA	Health Information Portability and Accountability Act
IOM	Institute of Medicine
ISAVE	Improving Social Determinants to Attenuate Violence
MUSC	Medical University of South Carolina
NIH	National Institutes of Health
USC	University of Southern California
VA	U.S. Department of Veterans Affairs
YAP	Youth Advocate Programs, Inc.

1

Introduction

Firearm injuries and death are a serious public health problem. In 2020, there were 45,222 firearm-related deaths (CDC, 2022), and each year there is estimated to be more than 80,000 visits to U.S. emergency departments (ED) for nonfatal gunshot injuries (Kaufman et al., 2021). In 2017, firearm injuries became the most common cause of injury-related death (Lee et al., 2022), and in 2020, firearm-related injuries became the leading cause of death in children and adolescents (Goldstick et al., 2022). Firearms are used in more than half of all deaths by suicide (CDC, 2022; Conner et al., 2019). Approximately 40 percent of individuals admitted to the emergency department for gunshot wounds experience relatively minor physical injuries and are treated and released from the emergency department, but the other 60 percent of nonfatal gun injury patients admitted to emergency departments face more severe gunshot injuries and are hospitalized (Kalesan et al., 2018). According to estimates from the U.S. Government Accountability Office, hospital costs for initial gun injury care total more than $1 billion a year, with costs associated with physicians' fees adding some 20 percent to that total and postdischarge care costing hundreds of millions of dollars more each year (GAO, 2021).

In 2013, following the Sandy Hook tragedy, President Obama directed the Centers for Disease Control and Prevention (CDC) to mount a research initiative, and CDC in turn requested the Institute of Medicine (IOM), now the Health and Medicine Division,[1] and the National Research Council to conduct a study. The resulting report, *Priorities for Research to Reduce the Threat of Firearm-Related Violence* (IOM and NRC, 2013), laid out priorities for a 3- to 5-year research effort. In 2019, the Board on Population Health and Public Health Practice of the National Academies of Sciences, Engineering, and Medicine convened a workshop that examined the roles that health systems can play in addressing the epidemic of firearm violence in the United States. The resulting proceedings, *Health Systems Interventions to Prevent Firearm Injuries and Death*, highlighted effective interventions that health systems can implement to address firearm injury and death (NASEM, 2019).

STATEMENT OF TASK

To continue the discussions from the 2019 workshop, Northwell Health and the PEACE Initiative requested that the Board on Population Health and Public Health Practice convene a workshop to gather ideas on how to integrate firearm injury prevention into the entire health care enterprise. The board convened an ad hoc committee and charged it with the following statement of task:[2]

> An ad hoc planning committee of the National Academies of Sciences, Engineering, and Medicine will host a 1-day public workshop to be conducted jointly with Northwell Health and the PEACE Initiative. The workshop will bring together firearm injury prevention thought leaders to explore how hospitals, health systems, and the health care industry at large can integrate interventions for firearm injury prevention into routine care for the purpose of improving the health and safety of patients and communities. The workshop will explore a broad range of topics including:
>
> - The state of evidence on health care strategies to reduce firearm injury and mortality
> - Barriers to implementing health care strategies:
>   - Patient/survivor perceptions and barriers to discussing firearm injury prevention with clinical team members
>   - Provider perspectives
> - Factors that facilitate the implementation of health care strategies

---

[1] As of March 2016, the Health and Medicine Division of the National Academies of Sciences, Engineering, and Medicine continues the consensus studies and convening activities previously carried out by the IOM. The IOM name is used to refer to publications issued prior to July 2015.

[2] The planning committee's role was limited to planning the workshop, and the Proceedings of a Workshop was prepared by the workshop rapporteurs as a factual summary of what occurred at the workshop. Statements, recommendations, and opinions expressed are those of individual presenters and participants, and are not necessarily endorsed or verified by the National Academies of Sciences, Engineering, and Medicine, and they should not be construed as reflecting any group consensus.

- How to adapt and implement public health and harm-reduction strategies across a variety of health care settings (emergency departments, surgery, primary care settings)
- The need for diverse perspectives in shaping health care firearm injury harm-reduction strategies:
  - Patient/survivors
  - Owners of firearms
  - Community-based voices (community-based organizations)
- Key elements of a health care industry road map for overcoming barriers to integrating harm-reduction and public health strategies around firearm injury prevention into routine care

OPENING REMARKS

The workshop began with opening remarks from the president of the National Academy of Medicine and representatives from Northwell Health and The PEACE Initiative, the two organizations sponsoring the workshop.

National Academy of Medicine

In his introductory remarks to the resulting workshop, Victor Dzau, president of the National Academy of Medicine, called firearm deaths and injury one of the most pressing health challenges facing the nation. From 2006 to 2014, the initial cost of inpatient hospitalization exceeded $6 billion or more than $700 million per year, a figure that Dzau said was likely much larger today (Spitzer et al., 2017). Prior to the start of the COVID-19 pandemic, firearms were one of the five leading causes of death for Americans under age 65, but firearm violence in the United States surged to record levels during the pandemic, increasing by greater than 30 percent. He noted, too, that firearm deaths and injury disproportionately affect certain populations, including those in urban areas, as well as Black, American Indian, Alaska Native, and Latino/a communities.

"There is an urgency to address this topic, and with an issue as complex as firearm violence, it takes a village to move the needle," said Dzau. "We need to address the whole spectrum of prevention and intervention with the full range of stakeholders." The health care system, and hospitals in particular, have an important role to play given that they see the consequences of firearm violence every day and because they can be strong partners in promoting community health, he said.

Since the release of the 2019 National Academies proceedings, the CDC and National Institutes of Health (NIH) have made efforts to restart research on firearm injuries as a first step toward preventing firearm-related violence and injuries. In addition, said Dzau, many other organizations, including the workshop sponsors Northwell Health and the PEACE Initiative, have continued to advance important efforts to address this issue. For example, Northwell Health launched the Center for Gun Violence Prevention, while the PEACE Initiative continues to support other organizations in their efforts to prevent firearm violence.

Dzau noted that this workshop will serve as an update to the 2019 workshop but with a distinct focus on addressing the barriers that health systems face to incorporate firearm violence prevention strategies into routine care and enabling the facilitators that can help them overcome those barriers. In addition, this workshop would focus on how health systems might incorporate input from important stakeholders, including members of communities affected by firearm violence, when considering how to overcome such barriers and enable facilitators.

Northwell Health

Michael Dowling, president and CEO of Northwell Health,[3] explained that his extensive involvement in the issue of firearm death and injury prevention began after the 2019 mass shootings in El Paso, Texas, and Dayton, Ohio. "As the leader of the largest health system in New York and the largest employer in New York, I felt that it was our responsibility—and the responsibility of all hospitals and health systems—to get involved in addressing what is clearly a public health issue," said Dowling. "Many people argued back then that we should 'stay in our lane,' that gun violence is not something that we should be involved in, but I argue the very opposite. We have an obligation to be involved and try to make a difference."

Northwell's response was to establish the Center for Gun Violence Prevention to organize Northwell's advocacy initiatives and help the health system focus on influencing public policy, public opinion, and elected officials, as well as educating the public about the extent of firearm death and injury.[4] Northwell has also held three national forums on gun violence and established a learning collaborative that now includes more than 500 health care professionals from organizations nationwide who are working together to make firearm death and injury prevention a priority. "If you are in the health care field and you are interested in health and public health, then you have to be interested in what to do about gun violence," said Dowling.

---

[3] Complete affiliation and titles for all speakers and moderators are available in the biographical sketches found in Appendix D.

[4] Additional information is available at https://www.northwell.edu/center-for-gun-violence-prevention (accessed August 10, 2022).

With a grant from NIH, Northwell in November 2021 began screening patients who went into its emergency departments to assess who might be a potential victim of gun violence. So far, the health system has screened thousands of individuals at three of its hospitals (Long Island Jewish Medical Center, Cohen Children's Medical Center, and Staten Island University Hospital), with plans to expand the screening to other hospitals. Dowling encouraged other health care organizations to not only do the same, but also learn more and implement violence intervention programs within the communities they serve. In concluding his remarks, Dowling said:

> This is a national endemic, and if you are working in the health care field you see the results of it each day. You see it in our emergency rooms. You see the results in our intensive care units. You witness the trauma that affects families and children, and the mental health and behavioral issues that result from gun violence. If we want to make our communities safer, if we want them to thrive, then this is one of the issues in which we have to be very forcefully engaged.

Jose Prince, vice chair of surgery at Northwell Health and surgeon-in-chief at Cohen Children's Medical Center, added a sobering reminder to the workshop. Several weeks prior to the workshop, a gunman shot 10 people aboard a Manhattan-bound N train as it pulled into the 36th Street station in Sunset Park, Brooklyn. Five riders were critically wounded, and more were injured in the following chaos. While that event made the national news, a little over a week before, in a less-publicized event, the ex-boyfriend of a Northwell Health employee shot her nine times in a parking garage as she left work, killing her. "Each of us can think about the impact of gun violence in our own neighborhood," said Prince.

The PEACE Initiative[5]

On the morning of October 27, 2018, a sole perpetrator carrying an AK-47 assault rifle launched an antisemitic attack on the Tree of Life synagogue in the Squirrel Hill neighborhood of Pittsburgh, killing 11 people and injuring 7, including first responders. Within 30 days of the deadliest attack in history on this religious minority community in the United States, more than 40 entrepreneurs from Pittsburgh, plus several honorary Pittsburghers including Bernard Rosof, cochair of Project M.D. of PEACE Initiative, gathered to discuss how to best respond to this attack. The answer, said Rosof, was to

---

[5] Additional information is available at https://www.peaceinitiative.org/ (accessed August 10, 2022).

work collaboratively with established community partners to help imagine, enable, facilitate, and fund fresh initiatives driven from an entrepreneurial perspective. The idea, Rosof explained, was to consider how the PEACE Initiative, a network of community leaders focused on addressing how health care relates to firearm violence in America, could identify key initiatives and help those community partners collaborate across their silos to move much more nimbly, measure results, drive actionable pilots, and then promulgate and use what works.

Convening this workshop, which is focused on how the health care community could come together to bring a perspective to firearm injury prevention that is driven by health care, was one of those key initiatives. Rosof said:

> We realized that this would most likely require a national collaborative approach that embraced regional and local health care systems, providers, patients, supporting health care organizations, community partners, and the communities in which they live. We understood that the way forward was to achieve an evidence-based approach to help evolve the mindset of our health care providers, systems, payers, patients, and community partners.

The PEACE Initiative is a small organization with big dreams, said Rosof, with the energy to support this effort driven by the haunting memory of what firearms can do to devastate communities. In closing, Rosof said:

> Our wish is that you all have the strength to move this [a health care driven perspective to address firearm injury prevention] forward in a meaningful way, to accomplish the goals of the workshop today, and then to take those ideas and move them from paper into practice, to see them piloted around the country, and to ultimately change the trajectory by finding the best pathways for success.

ORGANIZATION OF THE WORKSHOP

An independent planning committee organized the 1-day virtual workshop in accordance with National Academies procedures. The planning committee members were Andre Campbell, Erica Ford, Kayla A. Hicks, Kyleanne Hunter, Sandeep Kapoor, Peter Masiakos, Megan Ranney, Joseph Sakran, and Chethan Sathya. The workshop was broadcast live over the web, and workshop presentations were subsequently posted to the web along with links to the videos of the talks.[6]

This publication summarizes the workshop's presentations and discussions that occurred throughout the workshop's four panel discussions; Panel 1

---

[6] Available at https://www.nationalacademies.org/event/04-25-2022/facilitating-the-integration-of-firearm-injury-prevention-into-health care-a-workshop (accessed August 10, 2022).

discussed health care strategies to reduce firearm injury and mortality; Panel 2 presented barriers and facilitators to implementing hospital-based firearm injury prevention strategies in urban and rural communities; Panel 3 discussed collaborating with communities to improve health care system implementation success and destigmatize gun violence prevention; and Panel 4 explored a firearms violence prevention road map for hospitals and health systems. In accordance with policies of the National Academies, the workshop did not attempt to establish any conclusions or recommendations about needs and future directions, focusing instead on issues identified by individual speakers and workshop participants. Appendix A contains the references, Appendix B contains the workshop agenda, Appendix C contains the workshop statement of task, and Appendix D provides biographical sketches of the workshop speakers and moderators.

The workshop summary was drafted by rapporteur Joe Alper in collaboration with National Academies staff members Rose Marie Martinez and Dara Rosenberg as a factual summary of what occurred at the workshop, and the National Academies does not endorse or verify the statements.

2

Framing the Issue: Firearm Injuries and Health Care's Role in Depolarizing a Public Health Crisis

The workshop began with a presentation by Debra Houry of the Centers for Disease Control and Prevention (CDC), who provided an overview of firearm injury, prevention, and the role of health care systems in addressing this public health crisis. Houry said that her years as an emergency physician have made preventing firearm violence important to her, having seen firsthand the devastating toll of firearm violence on individuals, families, and entire communities. Firearm injury and death, she explained, have a tremendous impact on the safety and well-being of all Americans, with firearms taking the life of nearly 124 people every day, more than half by suicide. From 2019 to 2020, homicide rates overall increased by 30 percent, with firearm homicides increasing by 35 percent, resulting in the highest firearm homicide rate in decades, Houry explained (Asher, 2021; Johns Hopkins Center for Gun Violence Solutions, 2022). She noted that more people suffer nonfatal firearm-related injuries than die, and many of these victims experience lifelong physical and emotional consequences ranging from cognitive problems to paralysis. Moreover, the effects of firearm violence extend beyond victims and their families, affecting the community's sense of safety, affecting everyday decisions, and costing the United States tens of billions of dollars a year in medical and lost productivity costs.

While firearm injury and death affect people of all ages and in all communities, some groups are at higher risk. Racial and ethnic minorities, and particularly young Black males, have the highest risk for firearm homicides, said Houry, with rural and tribal communities, males, and veterans experiencing high rates of suicide by firearm. Most female homicide victims are killed by an intimate partner. Houry said:

Prevention efforts must consider the societal conditions disproportionately experienced by Black youth and other communities of color, and really address the root causes of violence. Violence is often the result of individual, family, and environmental factors that can accumulate over time.

As a result, she added, a comprehensive public health approach that targets risk and protective factors, with a focus on both short-term and long-term solutions, is critical to reducing community violence.

CDC's public health approach to preventing death and injury from firearms focuses on data collection and surveillance, research to understand and apply effective strategies, and cross-sector collaborations. To help communities identify the most effective strategies, Houry explained, CDC releases resources based on best available evidence on topics such as youth violence prevention and suicide prevention. These resources compile strategies that can help communities prevent violence, including firearm-related violence. Examples of evidence-supported strategies that Houry cited include reaching people at greatest risk through safe storage and hospital-based programs, improving the physical built environment through greening initiatives such as cleaning vacant lots and planting grass and trees, preventing future risk and lessening the harms of violence exposure through hospital–community partnerships and treatment services, and informing policies and programs that enhance economic and social stability by connecting youth to caring adults and activities, such as mentoring and after school programs.

Health care professionals and systems play an essential role in strategies to reduce violence in communities, said Houry. "Using a trauma-informed approach, we can improve patient–clinician encounters and lessen retraumatization," she explained. "This approach assumes that any person seeking services may have experienced traumas such as prior violence exposure, concentrated poverty, or racism." Hospital-based violence intervention programs are multidisciplinary programs that bring trauma-informed care to the patient while in the hospital and help deescalate violent situations. These programs can identify patients at risk of repeat violent injury and link them with hospital and community-based resources aimed at addressing underlying risk factors for violence, said Houry.

Houry then highlighted several examples of different types of interventions and strategies for reducing firearm-related violence. The first, Caught in the Crossfire, is a peer-led intervention that meets young shooting victims where they are, whether that is at home, the hospital bedside, or school (Becker et al., 2004). Evaluations found that 98 percent of the participants were not rehospitalized for violence-related injuries, and 90 percent of young shooting victims who returned from the juvenile justice system were not rearrested (Youth Alive!, n.d.). The second example, Virginia Commonwealth

University's Bridging the Gap Program, provides services to youth who have been admitted to the university's center for violent injuries. In this program, case managers connect youth and their families with the services required to break the cycle of violence and reduce the rate of reinjury and subsequent health care demands and costs often associated with violent injuries. CDC, said Houry, is currently funding an evaluation of this program.

As an example of how hospital–community partnerships can strengthen connections between the acute treatment of violence-related injuries and community assistance, Houry cited SafERteens (Cunningham et al., 2012). This emergency department intervention for youth uses motivational interviewing, skill building, and referrals to services to reduce the perpetration and victimization of peer violence, alcohol use, and dating violence (Carter et al., 2022; Roche et al., 2022). The Cardiff Model, another example, is a framework for sustained partnerships between health care, law enforcement, public health agencies, and other government agencies (Kohlbeck et al., 2022; Mercer Kollar, 2018). This multiagency approach to violence prevention, said Houry, relies on the strategic use of information from health and law enforcement organizations to improve policing and community violence prevention programs (Boyle et al., 2013; Levas et al., 2018; Mercer Kollar et al., 2020). The Cardiff Model has demonstrated a 42 percent reduction in hospital admissions from violence-related injuries and $15 in health systems savings for every dollar spent (CDC, 2021).

Houry said that clinicians can bring their expertise to discussions on the accurate, timely, and local data that are essential to understand inequities in violence, to guide prevention decisions, and to enable ongoing evaluation in health system-level quality improvement. Health care providers can also discuss the safe storage of firearms at home with patients. The safe storage of firearms can reduce the risks for injury by separating individuals at risk for harm from easy access to lethal means. Such practices may include educational counseling around storing firearms locked in a secure place, unloaded, and separate from ammunition as well as the provision of a safety device.

Another program focuses on emergency department counseling on lethal means and trains psychiatric emergency clinicians to provide lethal means counseling and safe storage boxes to parents of youth receiving care for suicidal behavior (Runyan et al., 2018; Siry et al., 2021a,b). Among parents who indicated the presence of guns in the home at pretest, all reported they had locked up their guns at posttest.

CDC's Injury Center, said Houry, relies on two key data sources. The National Violent Death Reporting System collects detailed information on violent deaths by pooling more than 600 unique data elements from multiple sources, including law enforcement reports, death certificates, and medical examiner reports, into a usable, anonymous database. The Firearm Injury

Surveillance through Emergency Rooms program supports 10 state health departments' efforts to collect and share nonfatal firearm injuries based on syndromic surveillance data.

CDC has also funded 16 awards for research projects to inform efforts to prevent firearm-related violence, injuries, and crime. These awards focus on identifying effective strategies to keep individuals and communities safe from firearm-related injuries. "Through this work, we will be able to better understand the characteristics of firearm violence and the effectiveness of interventions," said Houry. One project, for example, is looking at the effectiveness of a hospital-based violence prevention program for reducing risk of firearm-related violence and injury in adult victims of violence. Several other projects are collecting data and vetting interventions that have the potential to reduce firearm injuries in large urban communities of color.

Since 2000, CDC has funded 17 youth violence prevention centers that have partnered with communities experiencing high rates of violence. The Michigan Youth Violence Prevention Center, for example, developed community collaborations that resulted in the healthy development of youth in neighborhoods in Flint, Michigan (Kingston et al., 2021). Using six different strategies, the participating communities have seen a 38 percent decrease in youth assault-related injuries among those seeking treatment in the emergency department and a 25 percent decrease in youths' likelihood of being victims of a violent assault (Heinze et al., 2016).

Houry said that firearm injury and violence are substantial public health threats demanding urgent action to support and scale up intervention efforts in communities across the country. "We are committed to being a partner with each of you as we have collectively advanced this work to improve the health and safety of our communities," said Houry, and going forward, CDC will continue to work at gathering more timely and accurate data on firearm injury and death that can inform prevention efforts. For example, communities can now use syndromic surveillance data to drive changes and respond to hot spots.

In terms of what she sees as the most important questions for health care providers and community members on which to focus in the years ahead, Houry said she would like to better understand who the right people are to have discussions with about safe storage and similar interventions. While it might be clinicians, there is some research suggesting that law enforcement or a trusted partner might be the right avenue for having those discussions. Similarly, she would like to see research looking at the best way and best moment in a hospital setting to counsel about safe storage. Another of CDC's priorities is to look at how to engage communities to build resilience and decrease violence overall so that communities do not have to deal with severe violence. Houry said she was interested in how to best use telehealth, social media, and other interventions to prevent firearm violence.

On a final note, Houry said that hospital-based programs can access CDC research grant announcements via the CDC Injury Center website.[1] These solicitations are usually open to universities, hospitals, and state health departments, she said. CDC, she explained, uses a peer-review process similar to NIH's to make grant awards. If CDC receives a budget increase in 2023, it will have another funding announcement next year.

---

[1] Available at https://www.cdc.gov/injury/fundedprograms/foa/index.html (accessed August 10, 2022).

3

Health Care Strategies to Reduce Firearm Injury and Mortality

The workshop's first panel session on evidence-based health care strategies to reduce firearm injury and mortality featured three presentations. The panelists were Thea James from Boston Medical Center/Boston University School of Medicine, Rochelle Dicker from the University of California, Los Angeles, and Amy Barnhorst from the University of California, Davis. Following the three presentations, Frederick Rivara from the University of Washington moderated an open discussion with the three speakers.

Before introducing the first speaker, Rivara noted that despite the 25-year drought in federal funding for firearm research that resulted from the 1996 passage of the Dickey Amendment (Rostron, 2018), a number of individuals have spearheaded programs in which health care systems have collaborated with their communities to do primary, secondary, and tertiary prevention of firearm violence. These researchers, he said, have generated evidence that interventions can work and make a difference in reducing the burden of firearm injuries.

INVESTIGATING THE PIPELINE THROUGH COMMUNITY PARTNERSHIPS, INTENTIONALITY, AND COLLABORATION

To start her presentation, Thea James reiterated Rivara's statement that hospital-based violence intervention programs are absolutely effective. "They really do alter the life course trajectory for victims of violence and produce healthy, stable, productive, and high-achieving citizens. They also slow down the pipeline from the perspective of recidivism," said James. At the same time, she said, the results of these programs would be even better if they addressed with real intentionality the actual root causes of the pipeline, because they only slow the pipeline, not stop it. For example, a study that compared neighborhoods in Boston based on where the city's public transportation system had stops found correlations between lower income, premature death, lower education, lower life expectancy, and homicide rates. However, neither this study nor others like it investigated the findings to understand root causes.

In fact, said James, redlining policies, enacted during the 1930s during the Great Depression, created the neighborhoods that suffer from disparities in violence. Redlining refers to the historic practice of classifying neighborhoods according to how desirable they were from a mortgage-lending perspective, with neighborhoods with high concentrations of Black and low-income populations deemed "hazardous," as noted by the color red on maps produced by the Federal Housing Authority (Figure 3-1). The effect of redlining was to prevent Black and low-income families from having access to home ownership and the benefits of home equity for building generational wealth, which created two distinct socioeconomic populations that still exist today.

The way the effects of redlining perpetuate today show up in the social determinants of health and health disparities, including the distribution of firearm injuries and stabbings by hospitals in the City of Boston. Boston Medical Center (BMC), a safety net hospital that serves many historically

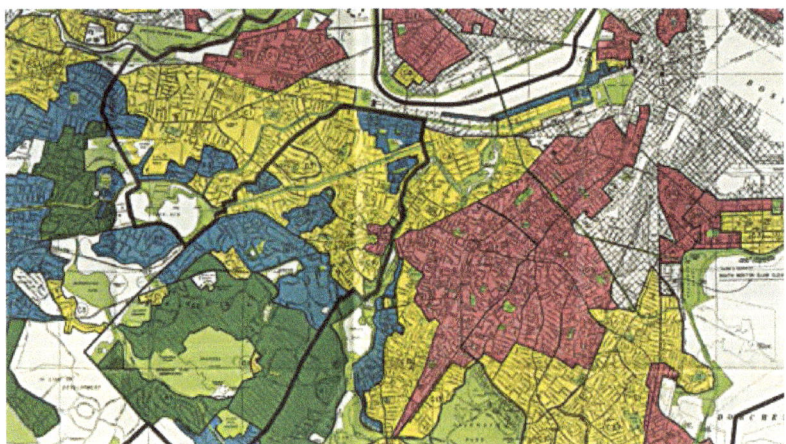

FIGURE 3-1 Federal Housing Authority's practice of redlining denied mortgages to Black and low-income populations.
NOTE: In the official maps, green areas were designated as most desirable, blue still desirable, yellow as definitely declining, and red as hazardous.
SOURCE: James presentation, April 25, 2022 (Nelson et al., n.d.).

redlined, disinvested communities, received almost three times the number of patients suffering from gunshot wounds or stabbings than the next hospital (Table 3-1). Similar patterns occurred during the COVID-19 pandemic, said James, with Black and Latino/a individuals from historically disinvested neighborhoods being the majority of patients seen at BMC for firearm-related injuries. James said:

> We all create programs to try to address the gaps [disparities] people have, but we do not eliminate these gaps, and when we do not eliminate these gaps, things do not really change in a very significant way.

The result, she said, is that despite having decades of experience developing models of care that address upstream drivers of health, there have been no changes in outcomes for health measures such as infant and mother mortality, diabetes mortality, deaths from cancer, incidence of depression and suicide attempts, and rates of homicides by firearms.

Beginning in 2018, James and her colleagues at BMC began asking whether the role of a safety net hospital is to perpetually fill gaps or to address equity issues. One realization they came to was that inequities are always present, but they are the status quo and look normal, so people do not investigate them. From surveying their patients who came from these communities, they realized they had two problems: access to care and distrust of the health care system, both among community members and the hospital's employees who lived in those same communities. James noted that when the COVID-19 vaccines were released, they were not deployed to the areas that everyone knew would be most affected during the pandemic, so her institution decided to create its own access program.

TABLE 3-1 Individuals Seen for Gunshot Wounds or Stabbing by Hospital in Boston

Hospital	2020	2021	TOTAL
Boston Medical Center	465	359	824
Massachusetts General Hospital	176	114	290
Brigham and Women's Hospital	83	67	150
Tufts Medical Center	57	69	126
Beth Israel Lahey Health	40	27	67
Boston Children's Hospital	7	8	15
TOTAL	821	604	1,432

SOURCE: James presentation, April 25, 2022.

By speaking directly to community leaders and having infectious disease physicians and pharmacists of color speaking to these leaders, they were able to answer questions about the vaccine and figure out ways to create better access for community members; these included establishing six vaccination sites around the city. In addition, BMC had data revealing hotspots and vaccination status at the household level. "We would show up at people's houses," said James. Data also drove operations at the six vaccination sites and enabled the access program to intentionally increase vaccine outreach efforts where needed. As a result, Boston achieved higher vaccination rates in the targeted communities than the state did overall, demonstrating that progress toward equity is possible with an intentional focus on addressing racial inequities.

From James and BMC's perspectives, the issue of equity comes down to economics and the ability of communities to thrive. To address this problem, her institution joined the Healthcare Anchor Network,[1] whose goal is to build more inclusive and sustainable local economies through hospitals being intentional about how they hire, invest, and procure. As an example, when a hospital in Massachusetts adds onto a facility, the state requires that 5 percent of the total capital construction cost must go to the community. BMC petitioned the state to invest its 5 percent in multiple housing investment initiatives. The state approved this request, and BMC has invested $500,000 of its $6.5 million in a private equity fund that will only fund developers if their proposal provides access to employment, green walking space, transit, healthy and affordable food, and affordable housing. The first result is Bartlett Place, with 323 units of new mixed-income housing units, some of which are available to own and some to rent, and a grocery store owned, rather than leased, by two community members. Greater than 60 percent of the workers building Bartlett Place are from the community. BMC established the Boston Opportunity System Collaborative, which is using a JP Morgan Chase Advancing Cities grant to address systemic problems that drive differences in economic opportunity within segregated neighborhoods while using vibrant social connections within those neighborhoods.

James noted that the COVID-19 pandemic prompted Boston Medical System to look at every aspect across its entire enterprise—operations, research, education, its health plan—to look for and investigate inequities. More than 80 leaders across the organization engaged to develop a comprehensive initial approach to advancing health equity. Six working groups representing all areas of the enterprise listed equity-based actions they intended to pursue over the next 12 to 24 months. The actions would address and investigate inequity-based disparities, with the intention of identifying the root cause,

---

[1] Additional information is available at https://health careanchor.network/ (accessed August 10, 2022).

implementing an intervention, course correcting, and closing the gap. BMC engaged patients to add context to the data. It conducted in-depth patient interviews to better understand the patient experience and identify potential drivers of the observed inequities. From these interviews, the working groups developed a long-term vision, an "institutional transformation," to advance health equity with clear strategic goals. It also created a prioritized list of 60 initial initiatives embedded across all areas of the system that are expected to produce results in the first 12 to 24 months.

James gave an example of a hospital's institutional change that has had an impact. The obstetrics/gynecology department engaged in a quality improvement project that found that postpartum hemorrhage was happening more often in Black women. Upon close examination, staff realized that this was connected to preeclampsia, which was resulting from the fact that it was taking twice as long for a physician to decide to deliver the baby for Black women. The treatment for preeclampsia is to give birth. As a result, the department has now standardized the decision-making process, eliminating subjective decision making and closing this equity gap. Robust qualitative research is embedded in this work to better understand potential factors that created the disparity.

Today, BMC's Health Equity Accelerator is working to transform health care to deliver economic justice and health justice across five areas: maternal and child health, infectious diseases, behavioral health, chronic conditions, and oncology and end-stage renal disease. James explained that this effort is progressing against a set of 2021 health equity priorities organized according to general clinical operations, high-inequity areas, social determinants of health, research and education, and advocacy, as well as talent, workplace, and culture. Informing this effort is its Equity Partnership Network, which includes a diverse, engaged group of Boston leaders and community members who provide guidance for BMC's equity- and community-based initiatives. The entire effort, said James in closing, is focusing on the root causes of inequities to mitigate firearm violence and other adverse health outcomes as much as possible.

THE AMERICAN COLLEGE OF SURGEONS COMMITTEE ON TRAUMA'S ISAVE INITIATIVE

To begin her presentation, Rochelle Dicker explained that the American College of Surgeons Committee on Trauma is responsible for verifying and setting standards and indicators for trauma centers from level I to level IV. She then noted that structural racism, the root cause of inequities that James spoke about, is the normalization and legitimization of an array of dynamics—historical, cultural, institutional, and interpersonal—that routinely advantage

White people while producing cumulative and chronic adverse outcomes for people of color. One of those chronic outcomes, she added, is homicide.

Similar to the map James showed in her presentation (Figure 3-1), Dicker displayed a redlining map of Los Angeles County showing the redlined areas such as Compton and Lynwood (Figure 3-2). She then listed the social determinants of health and health outcomes that arise as a result of structural racism stemming in large part from redlining (Figure 3-3). Structural racism, said Dicker, explains the association between race and social class. She also reiterated James's comment that without addressing the root causes of the social determinants of health, it will be difficult to greatly affect health outcomes. Dicker said:

> The physical environment and social determinants, along with behavioral factors, drive 80 percent of health outcomes, with 20 percent being quality related and access related, but many of us would argue that you cannot have access, really true access, without addressing the social determinants.

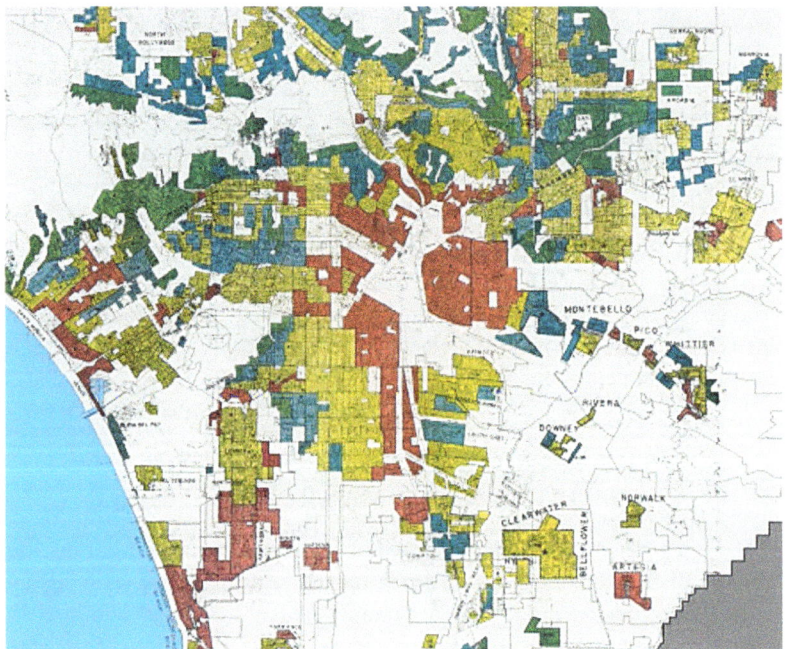

FIGURE 3-2 Federal Housing Authority mortgage lending map of Los Angeles County showing redlined areas.
SOURCE: Dicker presentation, April 25, 2022 (Nelson et al., n.d.).

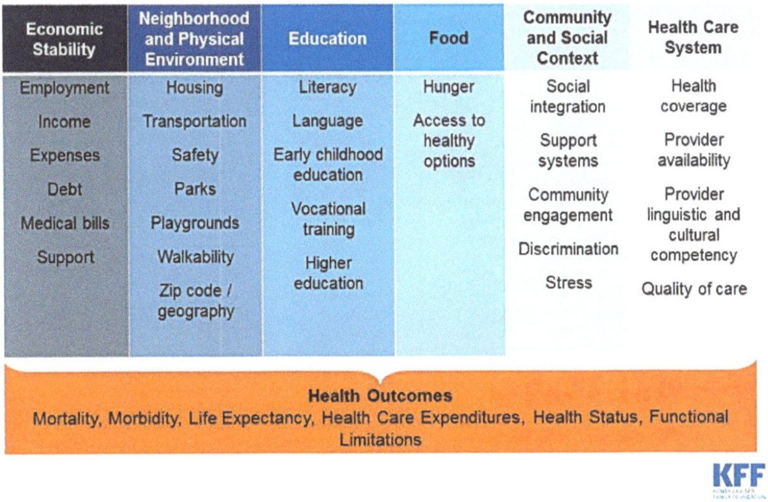

Economic Stability	Neighborhood and Physical Environment	Education	Food	Community and Social Context	Health Care System
Employment	Housing	Literacy	Hunger	Social integration	Health coverage
Income	Transportation	Language	Access to healthy options	Support systems	Provider availability
Expenses	Safety	Early childhood education		Community engagement	Provider linguistic and cultural competency
Debt	Parks	Vocational training		Discrimination	
Medical bills	Playgrounds			Stress	Quality of care
Support	Walkability	Higher education			
	Zip code / geography				

Health Outcomes
Mortality, Morbidity, Life Expectancy, Health Care Expenditures, Health Status, Functional Limitations

KFF

FIGURE 3-3 Social determinants of health.
SOURCE: Dicker presentation, April 25, 2022 (Artiga and Hinton, 2018).

To illustrate the connection between social determinants of health, violence, and chronic disease, as well as the interconnectedness of health and wealth, Dicker presented maps of Los Angeles showing the overlap of areas with elevated environmental health risks, homicides, unemployment, amputations from diabetes, poverty levels, and food deserts by neighborhood (Figure 3-4). She noted that even though 85 percent of physicians report that unmet social needs lead directly to poorer health outcomes, only 20 percent of physicians are confident in their ability to address unmet social needs (RWJF, 2011). Dicker explained that it takes a community at the table as a partner to address these underlying social care needs; addressing the individual social needs goes part of the way upstream to root causes, but going all the way upstream requires strategies that address laws, policies, and regulations that create community conditions capable of supporting the health of all people.

Prior to the COVID-19 pandemic, the American College of Surgeons held a medical summit on firearm injury prevention that included representatives from the American Bar Association, emergency medicine, public health, and other stakeholders (Bulger et al., 2019). The summit's discussions, which focused on different public health interventions and the role the organizations attending could play in preventing firearm injury, led to the American College of Surgeons Committee on Trauma establishing the Improving Social Determinants to Attenuate Violence (ISAVE) workgroup. This workgroup, in turn, developed

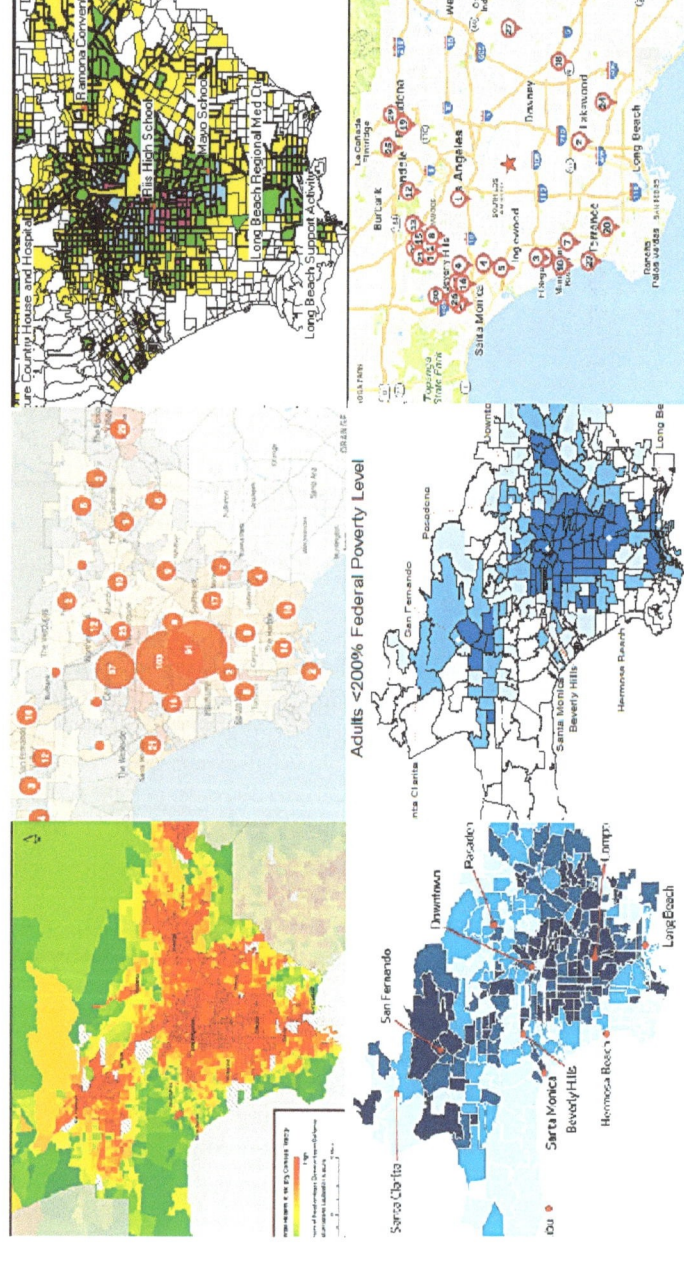

FIGURE 3-4 Maps of Los Angeles County showing environmental health risk (top left), homicides (top middle), unemployment rate (top right), diabetic amputations (bottom left), poverty level (bottom middle), and grocery store locations/food deserts (bottom right) by neighborhood.
SOURCES: Dicker presentation, April 25, 2022 (Google Maps, 2015; Google Sites, 2014; Hong, 2014; Stevens et al., 2014; Wezerek, 2014).

a set of strategies that trauma centers could employ to address the root causes of violence (Dicker et al., 2021). Dicker said that ISAVE has four main themes:

1. Develop a nimble curriculum for trauma-informed care.
2. Create a road map for investment in at-risk communities.
3. Integrate social care into the medical system.
4. Characterize the medical center's role in advocacy around the social determinants of health and equity.

Trauma-informed care, said Dicker, accounts for adverse childhood experiences and honors the fact that these exist in many violently injured patients. It also recognizes that many patients experience toxic stress resulting from prolonged, strong activation of the body's stress response system without having the counterbalance of supportive relationships to buffer that response. Toxic stress, in turn, negatively affects learning, behavior, brain development, and metabolic systems, and it can lead to the development of stress-related physical and mental illness (Shonkoff and Garner, 2012).

The trauma-informed care curriculum that ISAVE developed has six goals:

1. Identify and define trauma and its characteristics.
2. Identify and define the three *E*s of trauma—events, experience, and effect—and the four *R*s—realization, recognize, respond, and resist retraumatization.
3. Identify and define the different types of trauma that exist.
4. Identify the characteristics of a trauma-informed lens.
5. Identify the characteristics of trauma-informed care.
6. Identify how to render appropriate support.

This curriculum is based on the understanding that trauma is a difficult or unpleasant experience that causes someone to have mental or emotional struggles over time, and it is informed by the Substance Abuse and Mental Health Services Administration's six principles of trauma-informed care (SAMHSA, 2014):

1. Physical and emotional safety,
2. Trustworthiness and transparency that creates a space for human connection through up-front communication,
3. Peer support that integrates credible messengers,
4. Collaboration and mutuality that creates a model for respect and equitable care and responds to concerns,
5. Empowerment and choice that allows survivors to play a critical role in medical decision making and healing, and
6. Recognizing and addressing cultural, historical, and gender issues.

The trauma-informed care curriculum emphasizes a systematic approach. It starts with the idea that hospitals are trauma informed at a comprehensive level when hospital personnel practice trauma-informed care and exemplify the Beloved Community;[2] when trauma-informed care is integrated into hospital policy and physical layout—waiting rooms with water, tissues, and clean spaces to sit, for example; and when trauma-informed care is woven into the practice of all of the hospital's staff, including clerks, security personnel, administrators, and anyone else who comes into contact with trauma victims. The curriculum includes a segment on vicarious trauma, which recognizes that physicians, nurses, and other clinicians may experience vicarious trauma that can contribute to taking a nontrauma-informed approach with patients on occasion. Dicker noted that the curriculum includes a lived experience expert. Fifteen trauma centers across the nation will be piloting this curriculum during summer 2022. Data collection and analysis will lead to a second version of the curriculum that ISAVE will disseminate widely.

ISAVE has also developed a road map for investment in at-risk communities. This road map is based on a vision that health care centers will take an active role in altering people's life course toward a path of independence, including economic independence, and freedom from violence and chronic disease. Strategies to realize this vision include building external partnerships, providing opportunities for the community to have a voice, and retooling formal and informal medical education. Health systems can also leverage the Affordable Care Act's community health needs assessment and community benefits programs, as well as push for value-based care.

The third theme for ISAVE's efforts is to adopt a social care mission with two goals. The first is to provide tangible and working examples of the integration of social care into medical care. The second is to outline mechanisms by which hospitals can train, finance, and operationalize this integration. Along these lines, said Dicker, hospitals could design care delivery to integrate social care into health care, with hospital-based violence intervention programs being an example of a community-based violence intervention that engages credible messengers from the communities affected by violence as well as violence prevention professionals. Hospital-based violence intervention programs also provide long-term, culturally competent case management, provide links to risk-reduction resources, and seize teachable moments. Building a hospital workforce that can integrate social care into health care delivery and

---

[2] The Beloved Community, a term first coined by Josia Royce, is a global vision expressed by Dr. Martin Luther King, Jr., in which all people can share in the wealth of Earth. In the Beloved Community, everyone is cared for absent of poverty, hunger, racism, bigotry, prejudice, and hate (The King Center, n.d.).

fund, conduct, and translate research and evaluation of social care integration models are additional steps that can be taken.

Dicker mentioned two important resources: a National Academies consensus study report, *Integrating Social Care into the Delivery of Health Care*, that provides a road map for moving upstream to improve the nation's health (NASEM, 2019), and a primer on violence intervention programs for trauma centers released by the American College of Surgeons (Dicker et al., 2017). She also pointed out that the Health Alliance for Violence Intervention can provide training and technical assistance and will be releasing standards and indicators for hospital-based violence interventions.[3]

On a final note, Dicker provided a case scenario to illustrate why social care is needed. In this scenario, a 23-year-old male is in the intensive care unit with a gunshot wound for 13 days. On discharge, he is ordered to return to follow up 1 week after leaving rehabilitation. To a physician, the discharge process may mean writing the order and preparing a discharge summary, but for the patient it means juggling a variety of concerns in order to make it to that follow-up appointment. The key, she said, is to have cultural humility and understand how to measure value by listening to the community that is most affected by social determinants of health. She calls this social technology—when all the stakeholders are at the table being listened to in a way that can lift up people and enable working upstream.

THE BULLETPOINTS PROJECT

BulletPoints, said Amy Barnhorst, is a firearm violence prevention curriculum project designed for health care providers. While involving health care providers in firearm injury prevention is not the only solution to this problem, they can play an important role in addressing the multiple causes of death and injury from firearms. In fact, most physicians feel that counseling falls within their clinical responsibilities, and most patients, including firearm owners, believe it is generally appropriate for their providers to talk with them about firearm safety and injury prevention particularly when there is someone in the home who is at risk of attempting suicide. However, providers overwhelmingly say they need more information to hold these conversations with their patients and intervene appropriately. For example, many clinicians say that when they find out that a patient is at risk and has a firearm at home, they do not know what steps to take to mitigate risk. Clinicians also report needing more information about identifying patients who are at risk so that they can have these conversations.

Barnhorst explained that the BulletPoints Project got started when Marc Berman, a California Assembly member who wanted to do something about

---

[3] Available at https://www.thehavi.org/ (accessed August 10, 2022).

firearm violence but was tired of the partisan political battles over firearm legislation, teamed up with Garen Wintemute, an emergency department physician who runs the California Firearm Violence Research Center at the University of California, Davis. Together, the two came up with the idea of developing a curriculum for health care providers to teach them how to address the risk of firearm injury and death affecting their patients. Spurring this effort, she said, was the National Rifle Association's November 2018 comment via Twitter that "someone should tell self-important anti-gun doctors to 'stay in their lane'"[4] and the tweeted replies from the trauma and emergency medicine community talking about what happens in their lives and their work as a result of firearm violence. This outcry helped lead to the passage in California of AB521, which appropriated almost $4 million for developing, evaluating, and disseminating curriculum for physicians, surgeons, and other medical and mental health providers on firearm injury prevention in the health care setting.

The nine member, multidisciplinary BulletPoints team includes emergency medicine physicians, mental health professionals, a researcher with experience researching and evaluating large public health programs, and analysts with experience in evaluation, research, public health, and public communication. The team works with other clinicians, as well as experts who have experience in areas such as public health education and firearms research. The team has focused its curriculum on health care providers and health care educators, with the endpoint target being firearm owners, given that they are the people most at risk of firearm injury, suicide, and death. The idea has been to educate health care providers in a politically neutral manner using evidence-based materials. Barnhorst said:

> We encourage folks who attend our lectures and take our courses to keep their own personal politics, views, and or opinions about firearms out of the conversation, and instead focus on risk and the particular situation of the patient they are with at the time.

BulletPoints takes a culturally humble approach with an eye to the social determinants of health. The idea behind this approach, said Barnhorst, is for the clinician to put themselves in the shoes of a patient who may have a different political view, background, experience, and concerns while keeping in mind some of the social determinants of health that contribute to the risk of firearm injury. For example, people may own a firearm for a variety of reasons, with the most common in the United States being for protection. "So

---

[4] Available at https://twitter.com/nra/status/1060256567914909702?lang=en (accessed August 10, 2022).

while you may be aware that the biggest way to reduce risk might be to get the firearm completely out of the home," said Barnhorst, "oftentimes we have to work with folks using cultural humility and a harm-reduction approach to talk about what would be a good way that is acceptable to them to reduce the risk of firearm injury in their home and that they are willing to enact." For example, if they are not willing to remove all firearms from the home, a biometric lock box kept inside the home may be an effective compromise.

One thing the project team learned during the COVID-19 pandemic was the need for the program to be flexible as needs emerged. Before the pandemic, the idea was to hold in-person conferences and symposiums and attend grand rounds, but the program quickly shifted to an online platform and creating on-demand educational videos and recordings of program webinars, as well as focusing on its website as a place to disseminate material.[5] This turned out to be a good decision for the long term because it will leave a legacy in the form of a body of knowledge that will remain available to people who are working in health care and are interested in reducing firearm injury.

Material on the website is organized in sections titled The Basics, Clinical Scenarios, Interventions, and More Resources. The Basics section, for example, goes through some of the principles for how to counsel patients at risk of firearm injury in a way that is culturally humble and takes a harm-reduction approach. It also includes information about the epidemiology of firearm violence, the people it affects, and the disparities of who it affects, as well as information about firearms themselves for clinicians who do not have experience with firearms, laws relating to firearms and how they may apply to patients in the mental health system, the social determinants of health, and the principles of cultural humility.

The Clinical Scenarios section, said Barnhorst, contains scenarios that mental and medical health care providers may encounter with patients whose risk of firearm injury is elevated by the presence of a firearm in their homes. This includes scenarios on suicide, intimate partner violence, threats of mass shootings or mass violence, and dementia, all situations where a firearm in the mix may increase the risk of firearm injury or death. The scenarios provide the clinicians with a sense of how firearms may play a role as well as some of the steps that the clinician can take to reduce that risk.

The Interventions section, which includes links from the clinical scenarios, provides details on possible interventions as a means of empowering clinicians to ask their patients about their access to firearms. The interventions are presented in a risk-stratified manner, starting with safe storage, which is a good thing to counsel patients about if they own firearms regardless of whether or not someone in the home is at acute risk, said Barnhorst. They then move

---

[5] Available at https://www.bulletpointsproject.org/ (accessed June 30, 2022).

to interventions for riskier scenarios, such as temporarily transferring firearms out of the home at times of suicide risk or determining when a mental health hold is appropriate, and discuss how those steps might affect somebody's status in terms of being prohibited or not prohibited from owning or purchasing firearms. This section also discusses when civil protection orders are appropriate, so-called Tarasoff statutes, that require mental health professionals to warn a third party that they may be at risk of serious bodily injury from a client who threatens violence, and hospital-based violence intervention programs of the sort that James and Dicker covered in their presentations.

Barnhorst explained that BulletPoints uses a variety of avenues for delivering its content beyond its website and various lectures, presentations, and monthly webinars. BulletPoints has a newsletter and a blog featuring contributions from experts on firearm violence, and it makes extensive use of social media. It is also developing a continuing education course, sponsored by the American Psychological Association and the American Medical Association, and has created an educator's toolkit. She noted that medical schools from outside California have requested presentations, and she and her colleagues have conducted grand rounds at a number of organizations and medical societies across the country. The team has also published a number of peer-reviewed journal articles on the role of health care providers in suicide and firearm injury prevention (Barnhorst et al., 2021; Hoops et al., 2022; Pallin and Barnhorst, 2021; Pallin et al., 2022; Wintemute et al., 2022).

DISCUSSION

An audience member asked whether there are databases for temporary firearm storage locations. Frederick Rivara answered that there is a map of police stations, shooting ranges, and retail outlets for Colorado and Washington, and that there is an ongoing effort to develop a toolkit for other states to use to develop their own maps. Another audience member asked whether there are clinically validated risk and protective factor assessments for use with patient populations. All three speakers said that such instruments do not exist and would be difficult to develop because the risk of firearm injury and firearm death and psychological consequences of firearm violence are so individualized and varied.

Responding to an audience question about how hospitals can approach violence intervention with cultural humility, Dicker said there are two things that hospitals can do. First, educating people in a trauma-informed manner is essential, and second, integrating the community into the hospital and the healing process. "Once you start to do that, you see that the people who are caring for individuals pay attention, and they see the right way to go about addressing patients, not just keep them alive but help them to thrive," said

Dicker. It is also important, she added, to deliberately create a pipeline of providers who are from communities affected by violence and who already have the cultural humility that is necessary for this type of care. James agreed that trauma-informed care is extremely important because it is easy to inadvertently retraumatize people when a clinician does not understand that some of their behavior is a manifestation of trauma.

When Barnhorst was asked whether the BulletPoints Project was willing to share its curriculum with other hospitals, she answered, "absolutely yes." All of the content is available online with the goal that others borrow and use it. She added that because the project involved a terrific panel of experts to develop these materials, there is no need to reinvent the wheel.

4

Barriers and Facilitators to Implementing Hospital-Based Firearm Injury Prevention Strategies in Urban and Rural Communities

The workshop's second session featured presentations by five panelists: Rinad Beidas, University of Pennsylvania; Ashley Hink, Medical University of South Carolina; Scott Charles, Temple University; and a joint presentation by LeVon Stone and Sheila Regan, both from Acclivus. Andre Campbell, from the University of California's San Francisco School of Medicine, moderated a brief discussion following the presentations.

IMPLEMENTING FIREARM SAFETY PROMOTION PROGRAMS IN PEDIATRIC PRIMARY CARE

Rinad Beidas opened the session with a position statement, noting that she identifies as an implementation scientist. That, she explained, means that she uses insights from behavioral economics and implementation science to make it easier for clinicians, leaders, and organizations to use best practices to improve the quality and equity of care and enhance health outcomes. "I see implementation science as a way to advocate and amplify the needs of our communities and the pursuit of achieving population health and social justice at scale," said Beidas. She also said she is a Middle Eastern immigrant, mother, community member, and practicing psychologist in pediatric anxiety, identities that influence her perspective.

Implementation science is the scientific study of methods to promote the integration of various evidence-based practices, interventions, and policies into routine health care to improve population health, Beidas explained (Lane-Fall et al., 2019). She commented that addressing the research-to-practice gap including creating a plan for who on the team would be responsible for implementing each component, integrating the program into the electronic health record, and adapting the program for use as a suicide prevention program for older youth who were not in the age range for which Safety Check was developed (Davis et al., 2021a,b). Beidas and her colleagues also learned from community stakeholder input that the program needed additional adaptations to enhance its acceptability, appropriateness, and feasibility, and that it had to focus on suicide prevention.

Using the systematic adaptation process, the team emerged with a new program name, Safe Firearm, and logo that were crowdsourced using parents who are firearm owners (Davis et al., 2021a). They also learned from stakeholders that screening for firearms was less acceptable than having a conversation and offering cable locks to everyone as a universal strategy, which is how they now deliver the program. Beidas and her colleagues are now doing a large implementation study in Michigan and Colorado to test whether a less costly and scalable electronic health record–based nudge for clinicians reminding them to deliver the program is as effective as a more intensive and expensive facilitation (Beidas et al., 2021). The latter, said Beidas, is a more resource-heavy strategy to overcome implementation barriers. On a final note, Beidas explained that as part of a pilot prior to launching the trial, she and her colleagues are looking at signals for inequities to inform their approach to design for equitable implementation (Baumann and Cabassa, 2020; Shelton et al., 2020, 2021).

HOSPITAL AND COMMUNITY VIOLENCE INTERVENTION PROPAGATION IN THE SOUTH: UNIQUE NEEDS, CONSIDERATIONS, AND CHALLENGES

The experience of firearm violence, specifically homicide and assault, is different in the South relative to the rest of the nation (Figure 4-2), said Ashley Hink. She added that states with weaker firearm safety and responsibility laws tend to have higher rates of violence, which is true in her state of South Carolina, though this is not the entire story. South Carolina, with the fifth highest firearm homicide rate in the United States, at 11 homicides per 100,000 residents annually, bears a particular burden, with 85 percent of all homicides in the state committed using a firearm. Firearm homicides in the state, said Hink, have more than doubled over the past 10 years, from 229 in 2010 to 528 in 2020, and in Charleston alone, homicides increased 100 percent in 2020. "We truly have a major problem here," she said.

Homicide is the leading cause of death in the state for Black youth and young men, who are 7.4 times more likely to die from homicide than White youth and young men, said Hink, and firearm injuries are now the leading

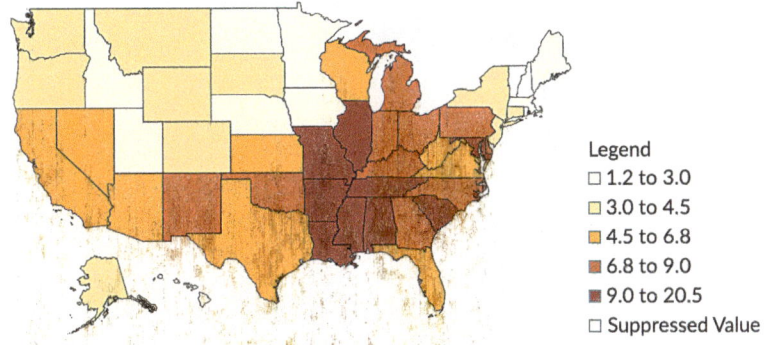

FIGURE 4-2 Firearm homicide rates by state per 100,000, 2020.
NOTE: Firearm homicide rates are age-adjusted.
SOURCES: Hink presentation, April 25, 2022; CDC WISQARS, 2020.

cause of death for children and teens in the state, with most of these injuries resulting from assault (Andrews et al., 2022). South Carolina has also ranked in the top 10 states for the number of murders resulting from intimate partner violence since data were first compiled, and in 2020 the state ranked sixth in the nation.

When breaking down risk factors at both the individual and neighborhood level, Charleston does not look that different from other urban, densely populated areas in the county. What is different, said Hink, is that urban and rural areas are both plagued by firearm violence. Poverty, intergenerational violence, lack of access to employment, and being underinsured, as well as an abundance of easy to access firearms, are some of the factors that affect rural areas as much as urban areas. The Area Deprivation Index—an index that pulls together aspects of income, education, housing, equality, employment, and more—shows this clearly (Figure 4-3) (Kind and Buckingham, 2018). However, she added, some regions of the state with the highest homicide rates are those with the highest deprivation (as seen in red in Figure 4-3).

The Medical University of South Carolina (MUSC), Hink's institution, is a level I trauma center for both adult and pediatric patients. In 2021, the trauma center treated more than 350 victims with gunshot wounds, 30 percent from the City of Charleston, 40 percent from the City of North Charleston, and 30 percent from the surrounding areas, which include some rural areas and small towns. In comparison, the City of Boston had 198 victims with gunshot wounds in 2021, a 28 percent decrease from the year before (Boston Police Department, 2022). What makes Charleston and South Carolina different, said Hink, is that there are no dedicated state funds for violence intervention, no use of American

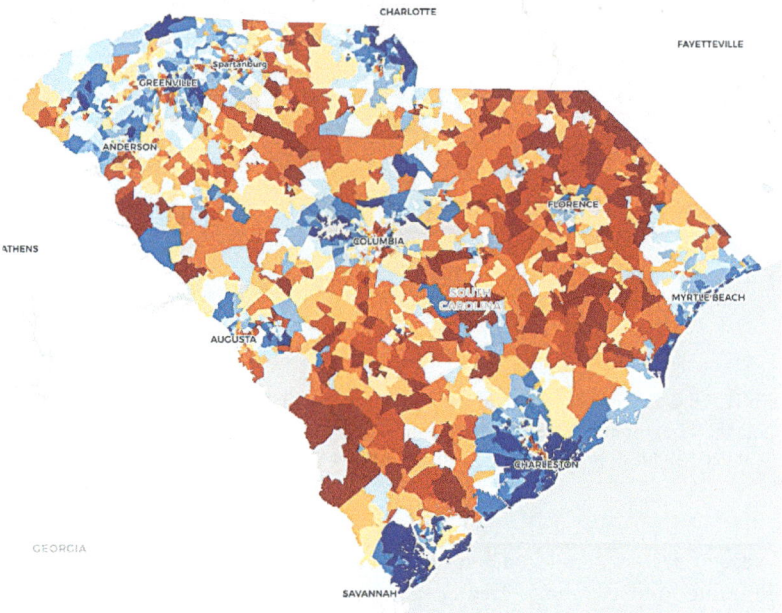

FIGURE 4-3 Area Deprivation Index for South Carolina, with red areas being the most disadvantaged regions and blue the least disadvantaged.
SOURCES: Hink presentation, April 25, 2022; Kind and Buckingham, 2018; University of Wisconsin School of Medicine and Public Health, 2019.

Rescue Plan funds for community-based or hospital-based violence intervention, no Medicaid expansion, limited city or county investment in violence prevention, and some of the least stringent firearm laws in the United States. Hink said:

> Not only are we struggling to find ways to actually pay for this work, but almost 70 percent of our victims of violence do not have health insurance, and so we see major barriers to care and access after they are injured and need ongoing care and support.

Nonetheless, her institution has implemented a hospital-based violence intervention program despite those barriers.[1] The Turning the Tide Violence Intervention Program got its start when the chair of the Department of Surgery, along with individuals in the Provost Office and MUSC, realized that the institution needed to do more to address this problem with

---

[1] The American College of Surgeons requires that all trauma centers must have an injury prevention program and meet specific requirements (ACS, 2022).

evidence-based strategies.[2] Hink and her colleagues identified allies and partners with shared interests and gathered local data on firearm violence in order to inform efforts and better communicate to the public the burden of firearm violence, and the need for and lack of investment in preventing firearm assaults and homicides. After securing financial support from the School of Medicine, the Provost Office, and the Department of Surgery, as well as using some state health department funds the trauma center receives for treating uninsured patients, Hink and her colleagues partnered with the Health Alliance for Violence Intervention (HAVI) to help start the program and train staff on violence intervention strategies. She added that program team members worked hard to integrate the program into clinical care and educate their colleagues and students. They also started celebrating the project and drawing attention to it to garner more support and resources to fund future efforts from philanthropic efforts and grantors (e.g., City of North Charleston Community Needs Grant and Dominion Energy).

Hink explained that the program's three frontline staff members were all born and raised in the Charleston area and have been involved in violence intervention work in their neighborhoods. In doing their work, they have support from injury prevention coordinators, as well as liaisons in pediatrics, pediatric surgery, and emergency medicine. In addition, her team has partnered with many local organizations to provide a wide range of long-lasting services and wraparound support for patients ages 12 to 30 with risks for, or injuries from, community violence in the Charleston tricounty area. Those services and supports include family support, victims of crime assistance, medical services, educational support, arts and music programming, employment and occupational training, mental health services, and a trauma resilience program. She noted that the program cannot provide the same level of intensive support for patients from outlying and rural areas, but it can provide some support and advocacy and connect those individuals with resources and referrals in their communities.

While that reduced level of intervention provided to patients in outlying areas may not be as meaningful in terms of outcomes that other hospital-based violence prevention programs have demonstrated, Hink said that many patients, no matter where they come from, report that they have benefited from the program and find the support and care they do receive is profoundly meaningful. One client, she recalled, said that the program "made him feel like a human being" after the program helped him secure a job, get his driver's license, and open a bank account. Since July 2021, the program has served more than 90 individuals and families and enrolled 42 individuals for long-term support.

---

[2] Available at https://muschealth.org/medical-services/emergency/trauma/turning-the-tide (accessed June 30, 2022).

One role the program plays, said Hink, is to propagate trauma-informed care, which involves changing the mindset of hospital staff in terms of what the victims of violence look and sound like and getting them to shift the focus from "What's wrong with you?" to "What happened to you?" This effort involved a significant amount of education and outreach to staff, students, and hospital leadership. It also involved getting the principles of trauma-informed care engrained in the medical school curriculum and into the fabric of the hospital community.

Hink noted that the City of Charleston is going through a revitalization effort that is changing the landscape of low-income housing, improving parks, creating green spaces, and renovating public housing units. Using data on violence at the neighborhood level, the Turning the Tide Violence Intervention Program focuses on areas that have the highest number of assaults involving firearms and partners with Youth Advocate Programs, Inc. (YAP) that have a history of propagating community violence interventions in those neighborhoods, in addition to other community organizations participating in community violence interventions. As a partner on a grant, YAP also coordinates with other organizations to provide wraparound services to youth identified by the school system, juvenile justice system, solicitor's office, law enforcement, and nonprofits as being at high risk of violence in order for YAP to act in a prevention capacity rather than as an intervention.

Advocacy as a means of raising awareness about community violence intervention is a significant part of the program. Team members have engaged with the community, given presentations to local organizations, and testified to, and held frequent conversations with, local elected leaders. Team members and other clinical staff have written newspaper editorials; participated in multiple educational events, grand rounds, and June 4 Wear Orange Day activities; and worked to introduce pediatric staff to other evidence-based programs such as safe firearm storage screening and use of cable locks. The overall goal is to become engaged in the community.

In closing, Hink said that one of the candidates for governor of South Carolina has included violence prevention and reduction strategies as part of their campaign platform, while a colleague of hers is running for Congress as a result of her passion for reducing firearm violence. Hink said:

> This is not meant to be an endorsement but to say that we have to be involved in advocacy in order to educate our leaders and to help propagate this work, especially in places like ours where it is not happening and is so desperately needed.

She also noted that following the epidemiology of violence shows that while certain populations and urban centers suffer a disproportionate burden, the U.S. Southeast has a profound disparity and lack of investment that is not matching need. Hink said:

> Many roads to eliminating violence disparities lead to the South, and our patients, our communities, and our health care systems deserve this [an investment in violence prevention]. We need to be propagating, supporting, and investing in evidence-based and evidence-informed violence interventions. It can be done, and we are excited that we have been able to do this work here.

TEMPLE UNIVERSITY HOSPITAL'S CRADLE TO GRAVE PROGRAM

Over the course of 4 years, Temple University Hospital went from treating just under 400 victims of shootings in 2016 to more than 850 in 2020, which Scott Charles said makes it difficult to feel good about the work he and his colleagues are doing to prevent firearm injury and death. Nonetheless, he added, he and his colleagues are determined to keep going and depend on the insights of those attending this workshop to inform their efforts.

Charles recounted how he came to be in charge of developing a firearm injury prevention program at a hospital after 17 years of working on community-based youth programs. In 2005, he had a chance encounter with Amy Goldberg, a trauma surgeon at Temple Health who was frustrated by the fact that the only time she encountered young people was when they entered the hospital as victims of violence. That encounter led to Goldberg tapping him to develop the type of initiatives he had been developing in communities across the nation. The next year, Temple University Hospital launched the Cradle to Grave program with the goal of deglamorizing gun violence through an immersive experience that would enable young people to appreciate the real-life consequences of gun violence without them having to suffer those consequences firsthand.[3]

The program brings young people into the hospital for a 2-hour presentation that includes discussions about the real-life events surrounding the shooting death of a local teenager. Young participants also visit the trauma bay, where medical staff explain the procedures they undertake to try to save a shooting victim's life. A classroom session also informs the participants about how gunshot injuries are treated, after which the participants engage in a series of reflective exercises that asks them to discuss the people they love, the people who love them, and how gun violence has affected their lives. Since 2006, said Charles, more than 14,000 young people have participated in the Cradle to Grave program.

---

[3] Available at https://www.templesafetynet.org/cradletograve (accessed August 10, 2022).

Charles said he is incredibly grateful for the way Temple Health has come to embrace this work as part of its mission, particularly given that many years and several leaderships ago, talking about the gun violence that surrounded the hospital was discouraged for fear that it would scare patients away and hurt the hospital's finances. "I am glad to say that my stubbornness has allowed me to outlast those individuals," said Charles.

One thing he learned about creating a hospital-based program during those years was the need to make people uncomfortable. By nature, he said, hospitals like routine and order and are reluctant to do things differently. As a result, it can be difficult for people to envision the role that a hospital can play in addressing the issues that exist outside its walls. He acknowledged that this attitude is changing, but lack of imagination is still one of the greatest challenges he and others face when trying to establish new programs. He also noted the emphasis leadership places on evidence-based programs, which he understands is important, but the idea that the next hospital program be largely based on the last hospital program is a threat to innovation. "Yes, we are here at this forum because the landscape is changing and more and more we recognize the link between gun violence and public health," said Charles. "But we are also here because we have not yet found the solution." In fact, he added, in places such as Philadelphia, with a rich history of violence prevention programming, the situation is worse than ever today.

Charles then recounted how in 2014 he received a phone call from a man named Wayne Jacobs who lived in north Philadelphia, a few miles from the hospital. Jacobs told him that in the decades since his release from prison, he had devoted his life to helping returning citizens reintegrate into society and trying to prevent gun violence. He was calling that day because he and others from his community were tired of watching helplessly as they waited for assistance to arrive for young people who had been shot. "Wayne wanted to know if there was some way for staff from the hospital to teach him and his neighbors how to lend medical assistance to shooting victims," said Charles. "I remember staring at the wall thinking, 'well, that is a crazy idea,' and then being struck by the thought that it was such a crazy idea that it just might work."

To see whether this idea would work, Charles approached Tim Bryan, an emergency medicine resident, a former respected Navy medic who had taught combat medicine all over the world. Bryan's reply was that not only could it be done, but also that it had to be done. Over the next year, Charles and Bryan met with Jacobs and other community members to get their ideas regarding a community-based first aid program. Two of the community members' concerns were that the program not be overly complicated and that they did not want to be shot by police who might mistake them for robbers going through the victim's pockets.

The 2-hour course that Bryan and Charles developed is known as Fighting Chance.[4] During the course, volunteer nurses and physicians work with local organizations to train residents to help save friends, neighbors, and family members in communities that are plagued by gun violence. Since its inception, the program not only has trained thousands of local residents, but also has been used to train violence interrupters, school staff, and law enforcement officers. In 2015, Fighting Chance was one of the only nongovernmental entities invited to the White House for the launch of the Stop the Bleed campaign.

Charles noted that the reason he told this story was that while it is important to listen to experts, often the real experts are community members who have not read a single article in a refereed journal and are often absent from the room when the experts conceive their ideas about what is best for the community. Community members, he said in closing, typically have the very insights that "we at large institutions will devote countless hours and endless amounts of money trying to gain," yet authentically integrating the community voice and perspective into gun violence interventions is one of the most persistent challenges to overcome.

ACCLIVUS VIOLENCE PREVENTION SERVICES

Acclivus' mission, explained Sheila Regan, is to support community health and well-being for Chicago-area populations that are at risk for violence and other negative health outcomes. Its vision is to provide all individuals with the opportunity to reach their full human potential regardless of past misdeeds, disappointments, or challenges that are influenced by internal and external causes. She reiterated Charles's comments about the importance of having an authentic community voice in the room that drives these programs. That has been critical for Acclivus as a community health organization that provides targeted health education grounded in public health methods.

Regan and her colleagues use data-driven interventions based on multiple data sets, including data the company collects and government and hospital data sets. They take a public health approach because public health is by its nature an intentionally interdisciplinary and inclusive framework that allows for respectful understanding of different professional roles across community-based organizations, health care institutions, government agencies, and law enforcement. "Everyone has a role in a positive and effective public health campaign," said Regan. A public health approach is also intentionally practical and efficient, easily digested by any population, and provides a role for each person involved.

---

[4] Available at https://www.templesafetynet.org/fightingchance (accessed on August 5, 2022).

All members of the company's leadership team are grassroots leaders who are committed to and invested in seeing positive outcomes for Chicago and who each have more than 20 years of experience in violence prevention and reduction work in Chicago. Though Acclivus focuses on Chicago, Regan noted that she and her copresenter, LeVon Stone, have also provided national and international trainings on hospital-based violence prevention programs. She also pointed out that Stone started doing this work in 2005 as a hospital responder and has since earned his bachelor's and master's degrees. As chief executive officer and founder of Acclivus, he can show the target audience that it is not how they start, it is how they finish, and that it is never too late to be the person they really want to be. Recently, she added, the company received a grant from the state of Illinois to provide violence prevention training across the state to different service providers.

The company performs its community violence prevention work at seven sites across Chicago. The primary services it provides are conflict mediation and case management with individuals who are at highest risk for becoming involved in violence. The hospital intervention program responds 24 hours a day, 7 days a week, to victims at five hospitals, as well as offering a variety of supported programs in the community that are complementary and support the same target population. For example, Acclivus supplies behavioral health services, and trauma-informed, culturally competent therapy provided by therapists from the affected communities. The program also has access to justice programs that connect individuals to legal resources focusing on reentry needs for individuals who are reentering the community from jail or prison and eviction prevention for people who might be experiencing housing instability. Regan and her colleagues also serve on various local coalitions and task forces focused on victim services, health care services, and public health issues. Currently, Acclivus is involved in 11 different research projects in partnership with five different universities. The company also provides technical assistance for 23 emerging grassroots organizations, with others coming on board.

Within 1 hour of receiving a call, someone from the organization is at a patient's bedside to support the individual and loved ones. Acclivus then networks with community-based resources to provide violence interruption and conflict mediation in real time anywhere in the city. In 2021, Acclivus served 2,628 of the city's 3,561 gunshot victims, along with 556 visitors at the patient's bedside. The latter figure, said Regan, was lower than expected in an average year because the COVID-19 pandemic restricted who could visit the patient. In a normal year, the organization serves twice as many visitors as patients. She noted that the median age of a person being shot is under 30 years, and while every population is affected by gun violence, no one is affected more than Black men (Giffords, n.d.; Kaufman et al., 2021).

DISCUSSION

Andre Campbell opened the discussion by asking the panelists how they fund their operations. Stone replied that most of the funding for Acclivus's programs come from the state of Illinois thanks to a line item in the state budget. Aggressive fundraising brings in additional funds from philanthropic organizations and hospitals. He noted that the organization has arranged for tuition reimbursement for program staff. When Campbell asked how they managed to get a line item in the state budget, Regan replied that it was through the organization's commitment to advocacy and building strong relationships with state leadership. "They know us, they know we are accountable, and that we are going to do right by every dime," said Regan.

Charles said that Pennsylvania has recognized what was happening in Philadelphia and elsewhere in the state and has begun to provide funds for these types of programs. However, sustained funding can be a challenge. Three years ago, for example, his hospital launched a 24-hour, hospital-based crisis responder program that receives state funding. The main issue, he said, is that funding usually only lasts 2 to 3 years, after which he has to look again for money to pay for the program. This is a particular problem, he said, for the grassroots or community-based programs with which programs such as his want to partner.

Hink explained that her program, the only one in the state, has had to piece together funding sources and look for funds every year, and she called out state leaders for not recognizing the needs to address one of the highest homicide rates in the United States. "Every day is a mass violence day in our state, and so we have to bring attention to and advocate for our patients and communities and say that this work is so important that it should be funded," said Hink. "This should be a line item everywhere, because we should care about people dying from violence."

Campbell then asked Beidas how she ensures that there is equity integrated into the various steps of the implementation subway. She replied that in the beginning, implementation science was not as explicit about the need to include equity, but in the past few years that has become explicit. To integrate equity her team first understands the potential inequities that might exist prior to deploying an intervention by identifying them and then tracking and measuring them to make sure they are not creating new inequities. They also deploy strategies to reduce inequities while doing the work. For example, suicide rates among Black individuals are increasing rapidly, so her team looks at that population when extracting data about who was receiving their program to see whether there were inequities in the way they were delivering the intervention. She noted that this work is led by Dr. Katie Hoskins.

Campbell asked whether any of the panelists' states had Medicaid waivers to enable use of federal funds to support these programs. Hink said that a few states have passed legislation to use Medicaid dollars to reimburse for violence intervention and violence intervention professionals. Her team has engaged the hospital's policy liaisons to lobby for support and Medicaid funding. "I think we will see expansion of that in some states," Hink said, "but we have got to get the conversation going to let people know that what is happening in [one state] can happen [anywhere]."

Campbell asked the panelists how they keep politics out of their discussions with local groups. Regan replied that "a true public health campaign is not about which [political] side you're on, you have to be on the side of health." She also noted that piggybacking this on Medicaid is important. Stone added that most of his organization's advocacy work with legislators is basically begging for funds. Being a community-based organization, he said, helps with the begging process.

5

Collaborating with Communities to Improve Health Care System Implementation Success and Destigmatize Gun Violence Prevention

The workshop's third session featured brief remarks by the three panelists and an extended discussion moderated by Marian Betz of the University of Colorado School of Medicine. The three panelists were LJ Punch from The T St. Louis and the Bullet Related Injury Clinic, Jake Wiskerchen from Zephyr Wellness, and the Reverend Michael McBride from LIVE FREE USA.

THE BULLET RELATED INJURY CLINIC

The T is a community of health working to reduce the effects of trauma in the St. Louis region, and the Bullet Related Injury Clinic (BRIC) exists as part of that work, explained LJ Punch. The BRIC serves as a resource to provide care for injuries to the body, mind, and soul that so many people are burdened with once they are discharged from the hospital after being shot and for the people near them who often also have bullet-related injuries to the mind and soul. *Bullet-related injury*, said Punch, is the term he uses to describe the constellation of physical, emotional, social, and spiritual injuries that occur after someone has been shot. The BRIC bridges the intense gaps in care that occur after interaction with the health care system and the long-term healing that is required in the weeks, months, and years ahead.

WALK THE TALK AMERICA: AT THE INTERSECTION OF GUNS AND MENTAL HEALTH

Walk the Talk America is a partnership involving Zephyr Wellness, an outpatient mental health practice, I.C.E. Firearm Training Services, and Mental Health America. Its mission is to reduce firearm suicides and other negative incidents associated with firearm ownership through formal education, outreach, and engagement with the mental health and firearms communities, Jake Wiskerchen explained. One influence on this program's work, Wiskerchen said, is the idea that all mental health professionals need to develop their cultural competence by familiarizing themselves with the literature pertaining to firearms, which must extend well beyond the gun violence literature and into the full range of firearm-related matters, prosocial and otherwise (Pirelli et al., 2019).

Though mass shootings get a great deal of attention, the more serious issue in Wiskerchen's opinion is the large problem of suicide by firearm that accounts for close to 65 percent of all firearm death and over half of all suicides. He noted that while 59 people, including the shooter, died in the Route 91 mass shooting on October 1, 2017, in Las Vegas, 67 people die by firearm suicide each day. This latter figure, he added, has been rising over the past few years. He also said that in many years, more police die by suicide than in the line of duty (Heyman et al., 2018), and that the rate of death by suicide in veterans is 1.5 times the rate of nonveterans when adjusted for population differences in age and sex (Novotney, 2020). Slightly greater than 70 percent of male veteran suicides are by firearm, while almost 50 percent of female veteran suicides are by firearm (VA, 2021). While the link between firearm access at a time of crisis and suicide has been well established, Wiskerchen argued that does not mean restricting gun ownership but rather restricting access during the time a person may be at risk of suicide.

Since March 2020, an estimated 12 million Americans became new gun owners, and Wiskerchen's concern is whether these people are trained in the use of their gun and whether they are storing it responsibility. The challenge to mitigating firearm violence is by talking to firearm owners in a confident, competent manner. While some people might argue that suicide is not preventable, he would like the firearms industry to be a partner in addressing the problem.

Today, about one-third of American homes have a firearm, and somewhere between about 40 to 50 percent of Americans either live in a home with a gun or own one themselves, said Wiskerchen. That number, he noted, varies by geography, but regardless, the percentage is high enough that mental health practitioners such as himself have to be competent about firearms because firearm owners comprise half of their potential clientele.

Walk the Talk America has developed fliers with a link to free and anonymous mental health screening tools powered by Mental Health America that gun shops can include in gun boxes or put on the counter where people might see them. Wiskerchen noted that screenings work, and they can help people become more attuned to their symptoms, be better able to talk to their practitioners, and be better able to monitor their recovery. He said that almost two-thirds of the 4 million people who have taken the Mental Health America screenings are ages 11–24 years, with women accounting for 73 percent of those who engaged with the screening tool.

Walk the Talk America also conducts training courses for mental health practitioners focused on firearms cultural competence. The training includes discussions about beliefs, behaviors, and activities of firearm owners, as well as an introduction to firearm basics and information about responsible storage and use of firearms. Concurrently, the organization also works to reduce the stigma of counseling among gun owners. "We want to demystify what the mental health process is," Wiskerchen explained. Work with gun owners also addresses red flag laws and attempts to correct misconceptions about those laws. These discussions also focus on language, replacing the word *safe*, regarding storage and ownership, with the word *responsible*. Responsible storage, he said, is defined as preventing unauthorized access to a firearm, whereas many firearm owners think *safe* means they are safe because they have guns all over their homes that may or may not be stored responsibly.

LIVE FREE USA

Reverend Michael McBride began his comments by stating that he knows and continues to believe that gun violence is preventable, and that the trauma that often lingers and even lives inside the bodies, minds, spirit, and hearts of so many directly affected families and communities needs to be addressed through tailored health approaches that are of appropriate scale and are culturally competent. For the past decade, he has been involved in leading communities across the country that are committed to organizing, building power, and educating people to appreciate that there are strategies that can reduce firearm injuries, particularly as they relate to groups, cliques, and gangs and the conflicts that bubble up from the neighborhood and result in interpersonal violence. In his view, it is possible to address firearm injuries without increasing the prison population and the historical criminalization of people of color.

McBride's work has used a racial equity and public health framework to address the problem using approaches such as harm reduction while trying to have the greatest effect on a community. He noted that in some communities less than 1 percent of the population can be producing more than 60 percent of the gun-related shootings and homicides, which means that it is generally a small number of people who are caught in cycles of violence and firearm conflicts, which have persisted over generations. "What we find, though, is rather than dealing with these conflicts or these individuals or families with a targeted approach, the approach has been a collective punishment framework," said McBride. The collective punishment framework, he explained, does not create the specificity or nuance needed to achieve a targeted universalism. Targeted universalism is the idea that there may be a universal goal, but because people live in different worlds, the interventions need to be targeted to reflect those different realities and lived experiences.

He noted that the strategies his organization takes differ depending on whether firearm injuries are the result of group violence, suicide, or intimate partner violence. This is important when these injuries involve people of color, he explained, because there are often unconscious biases that need to be examined by the deliverer in the public health system, either the intervention specialists or the interrupter that participates in these interventions. Often, said McBride, many people of color who come in contact with health systems and hospitals have already had a negative cultural interaction with a doctor, nurse, or security officer in the facility.

As an example, he said there are so many stories of individuals who have gone to an emergency department after they or a family member have been affected by a firearm injury and they and their whole family are treated not as victims but as criminals. This racialization of criminality is often left unexamined by many members of the hospital staff. Imagine, he said, being at the lowest point of your life, at the point of your deepest need, and you are feeling criminalized rather than being treated as a victim.

Part of the work that LIVE FREE USA does is to implement strategies across the spectrum of hospitals, law enforcement, and community benefit organizations that address the fact that people come into this system with unconscious biases that are unexamined. This is true whether that person is a recipient of system services, a victim, an employee, or employer. Moreover, these implicit biases often inform the level of service provided, the speed at which those services are provided, and even the bedside manner with which they are delivered. All of this is important, said McBride, because it is important when dealing with people who are living these very traumatic experiences that the immediate point of contact facilitates a pathway and a journey to healing, not criminalization or incarceration. "We believe that one of our first interactions has to be around how we help facilitate healing, not just for the person who is directly impacted, but their whole family network," said McBride.

Doing this requires appreciating that the line between victim and perpetrator is often blurred and depends on where one enters the life of that individual, he said. It may be, for example, that a person has been victimized by violence early in their life and never had the opportunity to be treated with the kind of care and tenderness that victims deserve. It may be that the person has never had the opportunity to experience a pathway to healing. McBride noted that many young people and families are experiencing death that is ubiquitous, yet they have no pathway or opportunity to benefit from a targeted approach that would address the trauma they have encountered.

McBride's hope is that as hospital systems become more integrated into the prevention side of gun violence they will take seriously the idea that their interaction and engagement requires a serious examination around the kinds of targeted strategies that are culturally grounded. In closing, McBride said:

> I do believe that hospitals, medical professionals, and others need to have a seriously culturally competent, dare I say antiracist, stance toward the ways in which the disproportionate impact of firearm injuries meets our folks, and they need to engage that work in a very structured manner.

DISCUSSION

To start the discussion, Dr. Marian "Emmy" Betz remarked that each of the panelists in some way touched on the importance of cultural competence or cultural humility and the need to be respectful and appropriate if the goal is to engage with people in ways that are meaningful. In that regard, she asked Punch to comment about what that means in terms of language and the words that health care providers, administrators, and programs use. Punch replied that the foundation at the BRIC is the concept of solidarity first, or what he calls radical generosity:

> The best way I find to connect with someone who does not know me, for whom there might be tension in terms of different life experiences, for whom there might be historical hurts and trauma, is by extending myself in a posture of generosity. I create a posture that welcomes trust, no matter who I am or what I am saying. I think that is more of a technique than a language.

Punch noted as well that the BRIC does not use the term *gun violence* because those are two stigmatizing words, and instead refers to *bullet-related injury*. The word *gun*, he explained, brings up intense feelings that come from the partisanship that arises as soon as a discussion turns to guns. "People either have gun positive or gun negative postures, and not many people are gun neutral," he explained. In addition, he said, as a trauma surgeon he has never seen a gun that shot one of his patients, but he has seen bullets, and bullets are the pathogens that create the physiologic, spiritual, social, and emotional reality of bullet injuries.

The term *violence* is even more problematic, said Punch, because in St. Louis, where bullets are endemic, he sees a significant population of people who experience bullet-related injuries in a way that had nothing to do with their social and economic status, their demographics, where they live or what they do, who they are, and what they wanted to experience that day. Instead, they experienced a bullet-related injury while driving their car, walking, getting on a bus, or leaving an event. While an unhealed bullet-related injury can fuel future violence, he said, the way it is experienced in the body and in life is often more subtle than that.

Wiskerchen agreed with Punch that the term *gun violence* is problematic. He also agreed with the comments that Barnhorst made regarding cultural humility and the importance of being humble and curious to ask questions and not make presumptions about an individual's perspective, whether it is a patient or a gun owner. Gun owners, he said, are not monolithic. It is not one culture that some parameters can quantify. In fact, even though he is a lifelong gun owner he did not consider himself part of the firearms community and culture until he joined Walk the Talk America in 2019. Because of discriminatory and judgmental peer pressure, he would not even talk about being a gun-owning clinician. He noted that even at its peak, the National Rifle Association only claimed 5 million members, while there are now as many as 130 million gun owners in America. Wiskerchen said:

> We need to keep that in mind and continue to remind ourselves that these individuals who walk through our doors are just that, they are individuals with their own unique experiences, and we need to be humble and curious enough to meet them where they are.

Betz then referred to the work that the American College of Surgeons has done with the involvement of surgeons who own guns, recognizing that there is a great deal of diversity within health care regarding firearms.

McBride said it is important to consider that many people in the Black community who have been affected by firearm crimes or incidents have had to bear the stigma related to gun violence not as a means of protection but as a means of criminalization. Often, he said, he shows up at a hospital, sits with families or young people who have experienced an injury, and witnesses the kind of service extended to them that is never tender or soft and instead is met with fear, distance, and often with a law enforcement professional standing next to them. For him, this says that it is important to enter these settings grounded by a framework of trauma, not a framework of safety, which he has observed is often the first type of interaction with a medical professional in that space. "It is rarely a conversation about 'are you well' but rather 'are you safe.'"

In addition, McBride said, there is often an interview with a law enforcement person while the injured individual is in the immediate aftermath of being injured, with family present in an agitated state, and there is concern about "safety" in the emergency department, not a conversation about the well-being of the family that is clearly in an agitated state. What he would like to see happen when encountering people at possibly the lowest point in their life is to have mental health professionals and deescalating professionals present who can help people process their grief, anger, fear, and pain, right there in that emergency department and before getting into other kinds of considerations. In summary, he said, not only is language important, but so are practices. "It is about the way in which we show up that speaks both verbally and nonverbally to families and community members as soon as they walk through the doors," said McBride.

Betz remarked that this characterization is so true, and that as an emergency department physician herself, she wishes she and her colleagues always provided a great experience. "I know for many reasons it is often not what we want to be, and there is a great deal of improvement that we need to keep pushing for," said Betz. McBride replied that there are experts in the community—faith leaders, violence prevention interrupters, public health interrupters, and others—who are experts in providing culturally competent care and who he would like to see hospitals engage in ongoing dialogs before a trauma event occurs. The idea, he said, is to widen the circle of expertise beyond the medical sphere and create an ecosystem of expertise that can help guide interactions with those who have experienced trauma.

Punch noted that the BRIC now has a chaplain on staff and that one of the greatest new experiences in his career has been to recognize how much fun it is to work in the community. "In community, everything we bring to the patient is transformed into a much greater whole," said Punch. He then raised the idea that medical professionals, including himself, do not understand the impact of what it means to have a bullet go through or be inside someone's body. This, he said, is an example of how important it is to listen to patients and be humble.

6

Defining a Firearms Violence Prevention Road Map for Hospital and Health Systems

Before introducing the panelists for the workshop's final session, Chethan Sathya of Northwell Health noted that the goal of the workshop was to focus on implementation and how to move from evidence-based strategies to actual implementation and practical solutions. Doing that, he said, is not possible without the community. The four panelists in this session were James Braxton of the National Institute for Criminal Justice Reform, Megan Ranney from Brown University, Tom Jackiewicz from the University of Chicago Medical Center (UChicago Medicine), and Rajeev Ramchand from the RAND Corporation. Rather than give formal presentations, panelists responded to questions posed by Sathya and commented on the workshop's major lessons. Firearms violence prevention road map highlights can be found in Box 6-1.

HOW THE PANELISTS BECAME INVOLVED IN FIREARM INJURY PREVENTION

To start, Sathya asked the panelists to talk about their background, why firearm injury prevention is so important to them, and why they believe firearm violence is both a public health and health care issue. Braxton said that he grew up in the Hampton, Virginia, area, had trouble in school, was incarcerated, turned his life around, and ended up working in the neighborhood in which he grew up and serving as a symbol of transformation to the young men in that neighborhood. After working for the Boys and Girls Club, where he engaged with families in Newport News and Hampton who had been affected by violence and the Reinvest in Supportive Environments for

> **BOX 6-1**
> **Firearms Violence Prevention Road Map Highlights**
>
> - Trauma-informed care is vital to improving patient–clinician encounters and patient outcomes and incorporating equity into treatment.
> - Firearm violence is a complex disease that can be prevented.
> - Firearm violence is a public health issue and a health care issue.
> - Implementation science should be used to strengthen the potential for success for hospital-based prevention programs.
> - Evaluation is necessary for the continuous quality improvement and expansion of gun violence prevention programs.
> - Improving the quality and timeliness of data can help to identify individuals' risk factors and firearm ownership in the population.
> - Hospitals can address social and economic issues that lead to firearm violence by engaging with the community.
> - The health care industry can address gun violence by systematically implementing effective gun violence prevention strategies across hospital systems.

Young People organization, a statewide juvenile justice reform initiative, he turned to violence reduction work with the National Institute of Criminal Justice Reform. This work is important to him, he said, because he has lived experience with gun violence and still experiences loss from gun violence both through the people who are close to him and the young people he mentors.

He knows, too, that health care plays a significant role in addressing gun violence because he was also a case manager in a hospital violence intervention program in Virginia. "I saw the young people that came in, I met their families, and I provided intensive case management for a year after that," said Braxton, continuing:

> I know what they need, I know what complexities they face in their community, and it takes credible messengers and violence interrupters who have lived experience to be in these spaces and help create solutions. That is why I am here.

Sathya then asked Braxton how often he feels that he is truly included in conversations regarding hospital-based or community-based programs that collaborate with hospitals. Braxton replied that before his work in case management, he had never heard of hospital-based violence intervention, even though he had been doing this work for more than a decade. He first encountered a program when he was working with two young people in the community who were shot and he was the first person at the hospital to help them. His thought at the time was that there should be a program to help these young people who come to the hospital and their families with resources. "It is typically not the guns, it is the circumstances around the guns and around these families and young people that lead to that," said Braxton.

Next, Ranney explained that she is a practicing emergency physician who also trained as an injury prevention researcher and worked on violence prevention long before she went to medical school. She took on the issue of firearm injury prevention some 15 years ago after a number of disturbing cases she saw as a resident and then as junior attending physician in the emergency department, particularly a young man who killed himself with his father's firearm. She noted that when she first started her injury prevention fellowship, multiple people, both within and outside of her institution, told her that although she could work on violence prevention, she had to be careful not to talk about firearms. After the case of the young man who killed himself, she decided she could not be silent and that is was essential to talk about firearms as a different source of violence, both self-directed and other directed, and something that could be prevented and treated the same way we prevent and treat other types of injury. "Making it a political third rail and not saying the word *gun* was not doing anyone any good," said Ranney.

Since then, she has been working with many of the people who spoke during the workshop to try to change the conversation around firearm injury and move it away from it being an us-versus-them problem to being a public health issue. As a public health issue, she said, firearm injury can be addressed with good data on risk and protective factors, with theory-driven interventions that reduce those risk factors and increase protective factors, and then with dissemination of programs that make a difference. Achieving this goal involves creating partnerships with community members, parents, survivors, and family members left behind. It also involves a great deal of work with policy makers, the media, and people who may not typically consider themselves to be part of public health.

Ranney noted that she has been fortunate not only to conduct funded research on firearm injury prevention but also to work as a cofounder of a nonprofit and serve on the board of the local Nonviolence Institute in Providence, Rhode Island, all of which deeply informs her approaches to this issue. Concluding her introduction, Ranney said:

> The biggest thing for me is that there is no reason not to talk about this disease in the same way we talk about any other disease as something that is both preventable, before it ever happens, using primary prevention, as something

that we can prevent after the first signs of disease using secondary prevention, and as something for which we have to take action after it has already happened using tertiary prevention.

Regarding interventions, Sathya commented that it is important to remember that despite there being a number of evidence-based solutions that work to reduce firearm injury, the health care industry has not been able to implement these strategies at large. "Of course the people who are listening today are passionate about this issue, but when you look at the health care industry overall, the implementation of these strategies is lacking in a majority of hospitals," said Sathya.

Jackiewicz introduced himself by noting that he has been at UChicago Medicine for 20 months, following more than 8 years as chief executive officer of Keck Medicine at the University of Southern California in East Los Angeles, and before that serving as chief executive officer of the University of California, San Diego School of Medicine. One reason he joined UChicago Medicine was to tackle some of the health issues affecting the approximately 625,000 people who live in Chicago's South Side community, 77 percent of whom are Black, 12 percent of whom are Latino/a, and 2 percent of whom are Asian. Greater than 50 percent of the community lives below the poverty line. Residents in the UChicago Medicine service area experience gun violence at a rate that is five times higher than the rest of Illinois. In the COVID-19 pandemic's first year, gun-related violence in Chicago increased by greater than 60 percent. Jackiewicz said:

> When I got here, I realized that if we were going to really make a difference in health equity on the South Side, we had to make the community safer, and with this level of gun violence, it was going to be impossible.

He noted that you cannot work at UChicago Medicine without seeing the impact of gun violence and what it has done to the community and to individuals living there, which makes it imperative to tackle gun violence and make a difference in the community. Making a difference requires focusing on economic issues, and for him that means hiring from the community through job training programs as part of the overall effort to address the root causes that others addressed at the workshop. He added that before going to Chicago, he read history books about the South Side and understood that many of the problems facing residents of the South Side are rooted in events that happened 100 years ago. "These are not new problems, so we are going to have to be really creative in terms of how we tackle this. Employment and creating opportunities is going to be absolutely critical," he said.

The final panelist, Rajeev Ramchand, said that his passion for addressing suicide prevention started when he studied for his undergraduate degree at the University of Chicago and volunteered to answer a suicide hotline. When he was in graduate school, the wars in Iraq and Afghanistan were raging, and because his brother was a Navy veteran, he could not turn his attention away from the emerging evidence about the effect of trauma on the men and women serving overseas. Wanting to understand the mental health sequelae of combat exposures led him to work on suicide prevention, particularly in the veteran community, and on evaluating suicide prevention programs, which to him, meant looking at firearms.

Ramchand said that as an epidemiologist, he comes to this issue with a passion for high-quality data. As a result, he is not only trying to understand the issues and the risk factors that others have spoken about but also working to improve the data infrastructure in the United States to provide more timely and accessible data on mortality, suicide risk factors, and firearm ownership in the general population. "If we can improve the data infrastructure, we can get to solutions, in my opinion as a scientist, much quicker and reduce the burden that firearms pose for suicides, unintentional injuries, and homicides," said Ramchand.

SUCCESSES AND CHALLENGES

Responding to Sathya's request to talk about some of the successes and challenges he has experienced, Braxton first explained that when he was the area director with the Boys and Girls Club and responsible for creating after-school and summer programs in the most deprived areas of Hampton and Newport News, gun violence was a regular occurrence right outside the club's doors. To address this situation, he first had to understand who the community leaders were, because even though he is a credible messenger and could connect with people in certain neighborhoods, he could not go into every neighborhood because he was a stranger there. Once he identified the community leaders, he built relationships with them, helped them understand what his intentions were, and listened to learn what their needs were in their neighborhoods. "You have to identify those needs and engage organically," said Braxton.

In his experience with hospital-based violence intervention engagement, he has seen programs that engaged well with the community and others that did not, and those that did not were largely stagnant and unsuccessful. Those hospitals that were successful went to community meetings and hired employees from the community. Taking that approach sends the message that the hospital is walking together with the community to create solutions and that it wants to combine the resources and assets it has with the creativity and authentic vision of those in the community.

Ranney, who has been working with the community-based violence intervention program in Providence, Rhode Island, for almost 20 years, has seen the program's funding increase and decrease and watched the number of firearm injuries in the community increase and decrease. One of the biggest lessons for her has been the importance of being relentless in advocating for the community and ensuring that her hospital's residents, security guards, trauma surgeons, emergency medicine attendings, social workers, and nurses are aware of and comfortable with the violence intervention program. That is all the more important, she added, for community-based programs, as opposed to hospital-embedded programs, because those community-based programs are invited into the hospital setting with the permission of the patient, thanks to the provisions of the Health Insurance Portability and Accountability Act (HIPAA).

Ranney said she has seen plenty of programs on firearm suicide prevention and discussions of firearm access and lethal-means counseling fail. As with violence prevention programs, suicide prevention programs tend to come in waves, where a particularly high-profile case gets attention and people get involved, and then attention fades and so do the programs.

One of the biggest successes and challenges that Ranney noted was around tracking actual data on both firearm injuries and what she calls firearm injury adjacent patients. Getting those data requires collaboration between the hospital system, the state department of health, and community agencies. "When I think about our biggest areas of opportunity, they are around expanding awareness and availability of high-quality data," said Ranney.

She noted that it is not the top priority of her violence interrupters to collect accurate data. Their top priority is stopping the cycle of retaliation and supporting both survivors and their families as well as the larger community in the days and weeks after an episode of violence. "We have to make it easy for them to have access to and track accurate data," said Ranney, who would like to see the same for firearm suicide and active shooter threats. She noted that her hospital system has received threats that are not always reported by the media, and she is not sure how well those are tracked on a national level. The American Hospital Association, she said, has been active in talking about active shooter threats, but it is something that needs more attention going forward to help motivate change. She also called for more accurate and culturally competent screenings and day-to-day interventions.

Jackiewicz said that active shooter threats have not been a big problem in Chicago or where he was in Los Angeles. Having said that, he acknowledged that he worries constantly about the safety of his employees. Last summer, for example, an attempted shooting occurred right outside of the trauma center. In response to growing concerns among the employees about their safety and feeling personally threatened, the medical center is installing bulletproof glass around the trauma center and adding metal detection systems that are more subtle than those in airports but that can still detect weapons. He also noted that students have been shot and killed in the past 2 years, which is unusual for the University of Chicago. In that vein, Sathya said that he has seen an uptick in momentum at Northwell Health to have active shooter training.

When asked about his successes or challenges with respect to implementation, Ramchand first noted that the National Action Alliance for Suicide Prevention has recommended that hospitals and health systems begin collecting postdischarge patient mortality and patient survival data as a patient-centered outcome. Researchers could use these data to test what is or is not working in terms of death prevention and firearm injury interventions. The alliance also called for standardization of external cause of injury codes and routine collection of them within the emergency department.

He then spoke about how he had certain conceptions about how to counsel lethal means safety for veterans and law enforcement personnel who are at risk for suicide until he spent some time at Camp Leatherneck in Afghanistan and realized those preconceived ideas were wrong. In an environment where it would be a signal that something was wrong if an individual did *not* have a firearm on them, it will take a different approach to help those individuals. Such an approach can only be developed by listening and learning from that community and having cultural humility, said Ramchand.

THINKING ABOUT EVALUATION

Sathya then asked Ranney to talk about how health systems and researchers can begin the journey of developing a framework to assist with evaluation in a collaborative manner that serves to support community organizations and produces the data needed to prove the effectiveness of these interventions. Ranney replied that building trust with the community and forming partnerships must be the first step. If community organizations do not trust that data are being collected for worthwhile reasons and not just to publish a paper, it will be impossible to collect the necessary data. It is also important to do the work, get funding, and help support people who are working on the frontlines of violence prevention, often at disturbingly low wages and with a lack of benefits.

Also needed, she said, are partnerships with organizations, such as the Centers for Disease Control and Prevention and philanthropic organizations, to provide funding to accurately collect and analyze the data. Partnerships with researchers and behavioral interventionists who can help community organizations move beyond constantly dealing with emergencies and lurching from one shooting or stabbing to another is also important. Ranney said:

> It takes space, time, and money to be able to move beyond that, to incorporate best practices, and to be able to think about what does the data show actually works versus what are we doing just because it feels good. I think that is a

critical question for us to answer, for the sake of those who are on the ground doing the work, for the sake of the hospitals that are investing the money, but most of all for folks in the community who are affected by this cycle of violence and its emotional and mental aftereffects.

As far as what hospitals and health systems need to do to get started on adopting firearm injury prevention based on evidence-based strategies, Ranney said the first and biggest step is to see firearm injury as preventable, perhaps even more so than diabetes or heart disease. The second step is to engage the community and experts. One place she sees health systems go wrong, despite their best intentions, is not drawing on the well-developed, evidence-based firearm suicide prevention resources that are available. Another mistake if the goal is universal screening is to not think about the potential harms as well as the benefits of universal screening. Ranney said that while the biggest risk for a hospital or health system is to not do anything, the second biggest risk is engaging with the community without cultural humility and using polarizing language, destroying trust in that community in the process.

TRANSFORMING COMMUNITIES TO PREVENT FIREARM VIOLENCE

Sathya asked Braxton whether he could share his thoughts about the critical components that health systems need to consider when developing a road map to move forward with efforts to reduce firearm violence in the community. Braxton said that there is no one answer and that ultimately most of the responsibility falls to the community. He added, however, that he would focus on alignment with what is already happening in the community. Unfortunately, he said, there is too little collaboration and too many siloed efforts that never connect with other programs. That lack of connection, he said, is enough to stop good work from going forward. Communication is the key, he added.

Beyond that, Braxton said it is important to ensure that top-level leadership at the hospital is aligned with the top-level leadership in the community and the top level of physician leadership. Leadership culture is important, too, because it can send a message about how important this issue is to the health system or hospital. Putting the violence prevention program in the hospital basement next to the morgue, which one program he worked with did, sends the message that the program is not important. In the same vein, getting community input in exchange for a $25 gift card might seem to be a good enough message to send to the community, but a better message comes from getting community input and creating opportunities for employment. In terms of addressing cultural biases that can exist, Braxton suggested establishing a diversity and equity board before doing anything else and ensuring that the board is involved in the entire program planning process.

Jackiewicz agreed with Braxton that alignment is critical. He recounted how when he first went to Chicago, he became involved in a 5-month long program that brings together city leaders to talk about what was occurring in the city that would make a difference. The main lesson he took back to UChicago Medicine was to improve his institution's alignment and engagement with the community and with other programs in the city. "It is the synergy we can create with alignment that is so important," said Jackiewicz.

He noted that his institution, with the help of community members, has assembled an extensive in-house team of violence recovery specialists who support trauma center patients. The specialists are integrated into the clinical care teams and work with community groups, like street outreach organizations, to provide wraparound support and connect gun violence victims with programs and resources that best meet their needs. The violence recovery initiative is also a workforce program. It is critical, he said, that UChicago Medicine hire members of the violence recovery team from the community. This allows the health system to provide individuals with a career track within the organization and a living wage and benefits, including a generous tuition benefit. Over one-third of the violence recovery specialists, many of them having personal experiences with violence, have returned to school for further education and training.

As a result of aligning the institution's economic power—it is the largest employer on the city's South Side, with 12,000 hospital employees and another 10,000 university employees—with its community-based programs, these programs are having a significant effect on reducing retaliatory violence. The UChicago Medicine trauma center's violence recidivism rate is under 1 percent (UChicago Medicine, 2021). Jackiewicz added that 10 years ago, the UChicago Medicine had a much different attitude about working with surrounding neighborhoods and largely avoided community issues. That began to change in 2018 when the hospital opened its trauma center. In the ensuing years, the hospital started to work with South Side safety net hospitals and federally qualified health centers to further promote and support programs that provide more primary care, behavior health, and other much needed services, supported by $26 million in state funding for first-year initiatives and up to $146 million over 5 years. The transformation of the health systems relationship with the community, he added, has gained steam as a result of the pandemic, which he said strengthened UChicago Medicine's mission to be an integral part of the community.

For Ramchand, another important first step is for a hospital or health system to understand the data about gun violence in their community and where the gaps in those data exist. "It is only through baselining that you can understand how you are growing and improving," said Ramchand. He added that not tracking a program and measuring improvement is a disservice to those working on the project, as well as a lost opportunity to build enthusiasm for a program that is working. It is also critical to understand the local culture regarding firearms as well as the laws that govern firearms in the community as a means of understanding the ecosystem in which the hospital operates.

He noted that he was part of an effort at RAND that reviewed state-level policies and their effects on a variety of outcomes. For example, child access prevention laws, which allow prosecutors to bring charges against adults who intentionally or carelessly allow children to have unsupervised access to firearms, were very effective at reducing suicide deaths among young people (Azad et al., 2020). States with stand-your-ground laws, on the other hand, had increased homicides (Degli Esposti et al., 2022). Ramchand said he hoped this type of research that evaluates the effects of laws will continue to produce insights into which types of laws can have the largest effect on the outcomes of concern. At the same time, it is important to understand how those laws affect people that worry about gun rights and about their effect on hunting, fishing, and other recreational activities.

Going forward, Braxton said he would like to see health systems engage in leadership advocacy training so that they can be effective advocates with state and local policy makers and help city leaders, for example, understand possible unintended consequences of policies they might enact. For example, a city might decide to demolish a decrepit apartment building, but that has the effect of displacing the people who were living in that building. Now, a teenager might have to go to a different school, one at which rivals predominate, and the teenager feels they have to bring a gun to school to protect themselves, an action that runs counter to an effective violence reduction strategy that was working in the community.

Jackiewicz recounted a story about someone he met who moved away from the South Side where she had been born and raised because she was scared of getting shot while walking to the grocery store. This common story highlights the need for violence prevention programs, health equity programs, investments in training community members, and other steps to be intertwined because unless people feel safe in their community, progress will be limited.

Ramchand's final comment was to not forget about suicide prevention programs for veterans outside of the Veterans Administration (VA) given that two-thirds of veterans never step foot in a VA facility. A national effort to prevent veteran suicide would involve private and public hospitals in the community and working with veterans with cultural humility and the understanding that a veteran might need a different intervention than a nonveteran.

7

Closing Comments

Joseph Sakran of Johns Hopkins Hospital concluded the workshop by first recounting his personal involvement with firearm injury. One autumn evening, he said, he went from being a healthy 17-year-old high school student to collateral damage and nearly being killed when he was shot in the throat with a .38 caliber bullet. For many years, he said, he never realized the power of his own story in mobilizing action on preventing firearm injury and death. Sakran said:

> Being able to tell your story, or in some cases the story of your patients or the story of your community, allows us to develop a narrative, a narrative that can change the hearts and minds of people from all walks of life.

In fact, he said that as trusted public messengers, health care professionals have a critical role to play in improving this public health problem.

Sakran then provided his highlights from the workshop. Houry, he said, provided a broad overview of this public health crisis, the importance of the data that the Centers for Disease Control and Prevention is collecting of firearm injury and death, and the need for researchers and communities to collaborate on finding solutions to this public health problem. James then discussed the need to understand how disparities have perpetuated over time and serve as the root causes of firearm violence, and Dicker continued on that theme by addressing structural racism, its connection to the social determinants of health, and the need to address unmet social needs to have a chance at changing the trajectory of firearm violence in underserved communities. Dicker also discussed the work that the American College of Surgeons is doing on trauma-informed care and the pilot program it is starting in 15 trauma centers across the country. The first session ended with Barnhorst's description of the BulletPoints Project's work developing firearm programs for health care professionals. "I think it's important to recognize that many of us often do not know how to ask or even answer some of the questions as it relates to firearm injury prevention with our patients," said Sakran.

The next panel focused on barriers and facilitators to implementing hospital-based firearm injury prevention strategies in urban and rural communities. Beidas started the discussion by addressing the importance of implementation science and providing some examples of how implementation science has been used to deploy firearm injury prevention programs. Hink then spoke about the hospital- and community-based violence intervention program her team created from scratch and the importance of telling the local story and demonstrating the regional disparities that are critical to the success of this process.

The highlights of Charles's presentation on the Cradle to Grave program described the need to be innovative and imaginative when approaching this problem, and to sometimes make people uncomfortable. He added that, perhaps most importantly, it is critical to understand that the real experts who understand the solutions needed are the people in the community. Stone and Regan concluded the session by raising the importance of authentic voices and linking the hospital as a true partner with the community.

The third panel, continued Sakran, focused on collaborating with the community to improve successful health care system implementation and to destigmatize gun violence prevention. Punch discussed the importance of taking a comprehensive approach to caring for an injured patient that moves beyond physical care to include emotional, mental, and spiritual care. Wiskerchen noted the important aspects of improving cultural competence and engaging firearm owners in a nonjudgmental way. McBride then discussed the importance of health care systems and professionals developing a culturally competent, antiracist stance in a structured way to change the experience for the victims of firearm-related injuries and their families. For Sakran, the final panel underscored the importance of stories, with each of the four panelists using their experiences and talents to tackle this public health problem and build the necessary trust in the community.

In thinking about all of the presentations, Sakran identified six core themes:

1. Eliminate inequity.
2. Engage the community.
3. Speak with authentic voices.
4. Display cultural competence.
5. Engage in advocacy.
6. Develop policies.

He noted that the role that health care professionals play in reducing firearm injury and death cannot be overstated; the two-tier economic system that is intricately woven into the foundation of the United States is evident in the analysis of education, law, and health outcomes. Sakran said:

> To effect maximal change, we must be able to understand and engage with the depth and breadth of the problem through targeted policy. This is critical because only policy can fix what policy created in the first place, and we heard today how for far too long, policy has been used as a tool of oppression.

Sakran said that as the nation faces dueling public health epidemics, it is now in a phase where it has both the opportunity and responsibility to eliminate health inequities that continue to decimate communities nationwide.[1] Honoring the indiscretions of the past, he said, begins with implementing actionable solutions to chip away at the existing inequalities so that the country can finally realize a healthy, equitable, and inclusive society. In thinking about his and others' successes as individuals, one thing remains clear to him. "None of us gets here alone," he said. "It is a collective group of individuals that allows us to be the best version of ourselves possible, and to move the needle forward in a way that allows us to be truly effective."

He noted that one of his colleagues, a fellow trauma surgeon, was shot recently, and it reinforced for him how difficult it is to care for injured patients, let alone when it is your friend and colleague. Sakran said:

> This just reaffirmed the fact that none of us are immune, and we are all part of the fabric of our community, and we all need to participate in the change that needs to happen in our own backyards to make community safer.

On a final note, he requested that when the workshop ends, that everyone ask themselves two questions: "What is your story, and how are you using your story, the story of your patients, or the story of your community to impact and change what is happening in your own backyard?"

After expressing his gratitude to all the speakers, meeting participants, the workshop sponsors, both Northwell Health and PEACE Initiative, and the National Academies staff who supported this tremendous effort, he offered his thanks to his fellow planning committee members. He then adjourned the workshop.

---

[1] As of August 11, 2022, the National Academies Forum on Global Violence Prevention is not currently active. Previous publications are available at https://www.nationalacademies.org/our-work/forum-on-global-violence-prevention.

A

References

ACS (American College of Surgeons). 2022. *Resources for optimal care of the injured patient 2022 standards.* https://www.facs.org/quality-programs/trauma/quality/verification-review-and-consultation-program/standards/2022-resources-repository/access/ (accessed August 12, 2022).

Andrews, A. L., X. Killings, E. R. Oddo, K. A. B. Gastineau, and A. B. Hink. 2022. Pediatric firearm injury mortality epidemiology. *Pediatrics* 149(3):e2021052739.

Artiga, S., and E. Hinton. 2018. *Beyond health care: The role of social determinants in promoting health and health equity.* https://www.kff.org/racial-equity-and-health-policy/issue-brief/beyond-health-care-the-role-of-social-determinants-in-promoting-health-and-health-equity/ (accessed September 1, 2022).

Asher, J. 2021. *Murder rose by almost 30% in 2020. It's rising at a slower rate in 2021.* https://www.nytimes.com/2021/09/22/upshot/murder-rise-2020.html (accessed August 10, 2022).

Azad, H. A., M. C. Monuteaux, C. A. Rees, M. Siegel, R. Mannix, L. K. Lee, K. M. Sheehan, and E. W. Fleegler. 2020. Child access prevention firearm laws and firearm fatalities among children aged 0 to 14 years, 1991-2016. *JAMA Pediatrics* 174(5):463–469. https://doi.org/10.1001/jamapediatrics.2019.6227.

Barkin, S. L., S. A. Finch, E. H. Ip, B. Scheindlin, J. A. Craig, J. Steffes, V. Weiley, E. Slora, D. Altman, and R. C. Wasserman. 2008. Is office-based counseling about media use, timeouts, and firearm storage effective? Results from a cluster-randomized, controlled trial. *Pediatrics* 122(1):e15–e25.

Barnhorst, A., H. Gonzales, and R. Asif-Sattar. 2021. Suicide prevention efforts in the United States and their effectiveness. *Current Opinion in Psychiatry* 34(3).

Baumann, A. A., and L. J. Cabassa. 2020. Reframing implementation science to address inequities in healthcare delivery. *BMC Health Services Research* 20(1):190.

Becker, M., J. Hall, C. Ursic, S. Jain, and D. Calhoun. 2004. Caught in the crossfire: The effects of a peer-based intervention program for violently injured youth. *Journal of Adolescent Health: Official Publication of the Society for Adolescent Medicine* 34:177–183.

Beidas, R. S., B. K. Ahmedani, K. A. Linn, S. C. Marcus, C. Johnson, M. Maye, J. Westphal, L. Wright, A. L. Beck, A. M. Buttenheim, M. F. Daley, M. Davis, M. E. Elias, S. Jager-Hyman, K. Hoskins, A. Lieberman, B. McArdle, D. P. Ritzwoller, D. S. Small, C. B. Wolk, N. J. Williams, and J. M. Boggs. 2021. Study protocol for a Type III hybrid effectiveness-implementation trial of strategies to implement firearm safety promotion as a universal suicide prevention strategy in pediatric primary care. *Implementation Science* 16(1):89.

Benjamin Wolk, C., A. E. Van Pelt, S. Jager-Hyman, B. K. Ahmedani, J. E. Zeber, J. A. Fein, G. K. Brown, C. A. Gregor, A. Lieberman, and R. S. Beidas. 2018. Stakeholder perspectives on implementing a firearm safety intervention in pediatric primary care as a universal suicide prevention strategy: A qualitative study. *JAMA Network Open* 1(7):e185309. https://doi.org/10.1001/jamanetworkopen.2018.5309.

Boston Police Department. 2022. *2021 end of year crime report.* https://bpdnews.com/news/2022/1/6/2021-end-of-year-crime-report-superintendent-in-chief-gregory-long-praises-men-amp-women-of-the-bpd-for-successful-effort-to-reduce-crime-in-boston-for-the-15th-consecutive-year (accessed August 29, 2022).

Boyle, A. A., K. Snelling, L. White, B. Ariel, and L. Ashelford. 2013. External validation of the Cardiff Model of information sharing to reduce community violence: Natural experiment. *Emergency Medicine Journal* 30(12):1020–1023.

Bulger, E. M., D. A. Kuhls, B. T. Campbell, S. Bonne, R. M. Cunningham, M. Betz, R. Dicker, M. L. Ranney, C. Barsotti, S. Hargarten, J. V. Sakran, F. P. Rivara, T. James, D. Lamis, G. Timmerman, S. O. Rogers, B. Choucair, and R. M. Stewart. 2019. Proceedings from the Medical Summit on Firearm Injury Prevention: A public health approach to reduce death and disability in the US. *Journal of the American College of Surgeons* 229(4).

Carter, P. M., R. M. Cunningham, A. B. Eisman, K. Resnicow, J. S. Roche, J. T. Cole, J. Goldstick, A. M. Kilbourne, and M. A. Walton. 2022. Translating violence prevention programs from research to practice: Saferteens implementation in an urban emergency department. *Journal of Emergency Medicine* 62(1):109–124.

CDC (Centers for Disease Control and Prevention). 2021. *What is the Cardiff violence prevention model?* https://www.cdc.gov/violenceprevention/about/fundedprograms/cardiffmodel/whatis.html (accessed August 4, 2022).

CDC. 2022. *Fast facts: firearm violence prevention.* https://www.cdc.gov/violenceprevention/firearms/fastfact.html (accessed May 31, 2022).

CDC WISQARS (Web-based Injury Statistics Query and Reporting System). 2020. *U.S. map of injury.* https://tinyurl.com/mta3jytk (accessed April 1, 2022).

Conner, A., D. Azrael, and M. Miller. 2019. Suicide case-fatality rates in the United States, 2007 to 2014. *Annals of Internal Medicine* 171(12):885–895.

Cunningham, R. M., S. T. Chermack, M. A. Zimmerman, J. T. Shope, C. R. Bingham, F. C. Blow, and M. A. Walton. 2012. Brief motivational interviewing intervention for peer violence and alcohol use in teens: One-year follow-up. *Pediatrics* 129(6):1083–1090. https://doi.org/10.1542/peds.2011-3419.

Curtin, S. C., M. Heron, A. M. Miniño, and M. Warner. 2018. Recent increases in injury mortality among children and adolescents aged 10–19 years in the United States: 1999–2016. *National Vital Statistics Reports* 67(4):1–15.

Damschroder, L. J., D. C. Aron, R. E. Keith, S. R. Kirsh, J. A. Alexander, and J. C. Lowery. 2009. Fostering implementation of health services research findings into practice: A consolidated framework for advancing implementation science. *Implementation Science* 4(1):50. https://doi.org/10.1186/1748-5908-4-50.

Davis, M., C. Johnson, A. R. Pettit, S. Barkin, B. D. Hoffman, S. Jager-Hyman, C. A. King, A. Lieberman, L. Massey, F. P. Rivara, E. Sigel, M. Walton, C. B. Wolk, and R. S. Beidas. 2021a. Adapting Safety Check as a universal suicide prevention strategy in pediatric primary care. *Academic Pediatrics* 21(7):1161–1170.

Davis, M., J. Siegel, E. M. Becker-Haimes, S. Jager-Hyman, R. S. Beidas, J. F. Young, K. Wislocki, A. Futterer, J. A. Mautone, A. M. Buttenheim, D. S. Mandell, D. Marx, and C. B. Wolk. 2021b. Identifying common and unique barriers and facilitators to implementing evidence-based practices for suicide prevention across primary care and specialty mental health settings. *Archives of Suicide Research October* 15:1–23. https://doi.org/10.1080/13811118.2021.1982094.

Degli Esposti, M., D. J. Wiebe, A. Gasparrini, and D. K. Humphreys. 2022. Analysis of "stand your ground" self-defense laws and statewide rates of homicides and firearm homicides. *JAMA Network Open* 5(2):e220077. https://doi.org/10.1001/jamanetworkopen.2022.0077.

Dicker, R. A., B. A. Gaines, S. Bonne, T. Duncan, P. Violano, M. Aboutanos, L. Allee, P. A. Burke, P. T. Masiakos, A. Hink, D. A. Kuhls, D. Shapiro, and R. M. Stewart. 2017. Violence intervention programs: A primer for developing a comprehensive program for trauma centers. *Bulletin of the American College of Surgeons* 102(10):20–29.

Dicker, R. A., A. Thomas, E. M. Bulger, R. M. Stewart, S. Bonne, T. A. Dechert, R. Smith, A. Love-Craighead, F. Dreier, M. Kotagal, T. Kozyckyj, and H. Michaels. 2021. Strategies for trauma centers to address the root causes of violence: Recommendations from the Improving Social Determinants to Attenuate Violence (ISAVE) workgroup of the American College of Surgeons Committee on Trauma. *Journal of the American College of Surgeons* 233(3):471–478. e471.

Fernandez, M. E., G. A. ten Hoor, S. van Lieshout, S. A. Rodriguez, R. S. Beidas, G. Parcel, R. A. C. Ruiter, C. M. Markham, and G. Kok. 2019. Implementation mapping: Using intervention mapping to develop implementation strategies. *Frontiers in Public Health* 7.

GAO (Government Accountability Office). 2021. *Firearm injuries: Health care service needs and costs*. Washington, DC: U.S. Government Accountability Office.

Giffords. n.d. *Statistics*. https://giffords.org/lawcenter/gun-violence-statistics/ (accessed August 11, 2022).

Goldstick, J. E., R. M. Cunningham, and P. M. Carter. 2022. Current causes of death in children and adolescents in the United States. *New England Journal of Medicine* 386(20):1955–1956. https://doi.org/10.1056/NEJMc2201761.

Google Maps. 2015. Trader Joe's CA (Los Angeles). https://www.google.com/maps/d/u/0/viewer?hl=en_US&mid=1rsmPsVI3HcG6rLtggj0MPTmPmh8&ll=33.92903099390304%2C-118.09479792655391&z=10 (accessed August 10, 2022).

Google Sites. 2014. *South Los Angeles jobs*. https://sites.google.com/site/southlosangeles111/jobs (accessed August 10, 2022).

Heinze, J. E., T. M. Reischl, M. Bai, J. S. Roche, S. Morrel-Samuels, R. M. Cunningham, and M. A. Zimmerman. 2016. A comprehensive prevention approach to reducing assault offenses and assault injuries among youth. *Prevention Science* 17(2):167–176.

Heyman, M., J. Dill, and R. Douglas. 2018. The Ruderman white paper on mental health and suicide of first responders. https://www.themarshallproject.org/2017/10/03/it-s-time-we-talk-about-police-suicide (accessed August 9, 2022).

Hong, S. 2014. UCLA, EDF identify opportunities to curb climate pollution, spur clean energy jobs in L.A. https://newsroom.ucla.edu/releases/ucla-edf-identify-opportunities-to-curb-climate-pollution-spur-clean-energy-jobs-in-l-a (accessed August 10, 2022).

Hoops, K., J. Fahimi, L. Khoeur, C. Studenmund, C. Barber, A. Barnhorst, M. E. Betz, C. K. Crifasi, J. A. Davis, W. Dewispelaere, L. Fisher, P. K. Howard, A. Ketterer, E. Marcolini, P. S. Nestadt, J. Rozel, J. A. Simonetti, S. Spitzer, M. Victoroff, B. H. Williams, L. Howley, and M. L. Ranney. 2022. Consensus-driven priorities for firearm injury education among medical professionals. *Academic Medicine* 97(1):93–104.

IOM and NRC (Institute of Medicine and National Research Council). 2013. *Priorities for research to reduce the threat of firearm-related violence.* Washington, DC: The National Academies Press. https://doi.org/10.17226/18319.

Ip, E. H., R. Wasserman, and S. Barkin. 2011. Comparison of intraclass correlation coefficient estimates and standard errors between using cross-sectional and repeated measurement data: The Safety Check cluster randomized trial. *Contemporary Clinical Trials* 32(2):225–232.

Johns Hopkins Center for Gun Violence Solutions. 2022. *A year in review 2020 gun deaths in the U.S.* https://publichealth.jhu.edu/gun-violence-solutions (accessed August 10, 2022).

Kalesan, B., Y. Zuo, Z. Xuan, M. B. Siegel, J. Fagan, C. Branas, and S. Galea. 2018. A multi-decade joinpoint analysis of firearm injury severity. *Trauma Surgery & Acute Care Open* 3(1):e000139.

Kaufman, E. J., D. J. Wiebe, R. A. Xiong, C. N. Morrison, M. J. Seamon, and M. K. Delgado. 2021. Epidemiologic trends in fatal and nonfatal firearm injuries in the US, 2009-2017. *JAMA Internal Medicine* 181(2):237–244. https://doi.org/10.1001/jamainternmed.2020.6696.

Kind, A. J. H., and W. R. Buckingham. 2018. Making neighborhood-disadvantage metrics accessible— the neighborhood atlas. *New England Journal of Medicine* 378(26):2456–2458. https://doi.org/10.1056/NEJMp1802313 AND University of Wisconsin School of Medicine Public Health. 2015 Area Deprivation Index v2.0. Downloaded from https://www.neighborhoodatlas.medicine.wisc.edu.

Kingston, B. E., M. A. Zimmerman, M. L. Wendel, D. Gorman-Smith, E. Wright-Kelly, S. A. Mattson, and A.-R. T. Trudeau. 2021. Developing and implementing community-level strategies for preventing youth violence in the United States. *American Journal of Public Health* 111(S1):S20-S24.

Kohlbeck, S., M. Levas, J. Hernandez-Meier, and S. Hargarten. 2022. Implementing the Cardiff Model for violence prevention: Using the diffusion of innovation theory to understand facilitators and barriers to implementation. *Injury Prevention* 28(1):49.

Lane-Fall, M. B., G. M. Curran, and R. S. Beidas. 2019. Scoping implementation science for the beginner: Locating yourself on the "subway line" of translational research. *BMC Medical Research Methodology* 19(1):133.

Lee, L. K., K. Douglas, and D. Hemenway. 2022. Crossing lines—a change in the leading cause of death among U.S. Children. *New England Journal of Medicine* 386(16):1485–1487. https://doi.org/10.1056/NEJMp2200169.

Levas, M. N., J. L. Hernandez-Meier, S. Kohlbeck, N. Piotrowski, and S. Hargarten. 2018. Integrating population health data on violence into the emergency department: A feasibility and implementation study. *Journal of Trauma Nursing* 25(3):149–158.

Mercer Kollar, L. M., S. A. Sumner, S. F. Jacoby, and G. Ridgeway. 2018. Cardiff Model toolkit community guidance for violence prevention. https://www.cdc.gov/violenceprevention/pdf/cardiffmodel/cardiff-toolkit508.pdf (accessed June 30, 2022).

Mercer Kollar, L. M., S. A. Sumner, B. Bartholow, D. T. Wu, J. C. Moore, E. W. Mays, E. V. Atkins, D. A. Fraser, C. E. Flood, and J. P. Shepherd. 2020. Building capacity for injury prevention: A process evaluation of a replication of the Cardiff violence prevention programme in the southeastern USA. *Injury Prevention* 26(3):221–228.

Monuteaux, M. C., D. Azrael, and M. Miller. 2019. Association of increased safe household firearm storage with firearm suicide and unintentional death among US youths. *Journal of the American Medical Association Pediatrics* 173(7):657–662.

NASEM (National Acadmies of Sciences, Engineering, and Medicine). 2019. *Health systems interventions to prevent firearm injuries and death: Proceedings of a workshop.* Edited by J. Alper, M. French, and A. Wojtowicz. Washington, DC: The National Academies Press.

Nelson, R. K., L. Winling, R. Marciano, and N. Connolly. n.d. Mapping inequality. *American Panorama.* https://dsl.richmond.edu/panorama/redlining (accessed August 10, 2022).

Novotney, A. 2020. *Stopping military and veteran suicides.* https://www.apa.org/monitor/2020/01/ce-corner-suicide (accessed August 11, 2022).

Pallin, R., and A. Barnhorst. 2021. Clinical strategies for reducing firearm suicide. *Injury Epidemiology* 8(1):57.

Pallin, R., S. Teasdale, A. Agnoli, S. Spitzer, R. Asif-Sattar, G. J. Wintemute, and A. Barnhorst. 2022. Talking about firearm injury prevention with patients: A survey of medical residents. *BMC Medical Education* 22(1):14.

Paltiel, A. D., J. L. Schwartz, A. Zheng, and R. P. Walensky. 2021. Clinical outcomes of a COVID-19 vaccine: Implementation over efficacy. *Health Affairs* 40(1):42–52.

Pirelli, G., H. Wechsler, and R. J. Cramer. 2019. *The behavioral science of firearms: Implications for mental health, law and policy.* Oxford, UK: Oxford University Press.

Proctor, E. K., and E. Geng. 2021. A new lane for science. *Science* 374(6568):659.

Roche, J. S., M. L. Philyaw-Kotov, E. Sigel, A. B. Eisman, G. Tzilos Wernette, K. Resnicow, P. M. Carter, R. M. Cunningham, and M. A. Walton. 2022. Implementation of a youth violence prevention programme in primary care. *Injury Prevention* 28(3):231–237.

Rostron, A. 2018. The Dickey amendment on federal funding for research on gun violence: A legal dissection. *American Journal of Public Health* 108(7):865–867.

Runyan, C. W., A. Brooks-Russell, G. Tung, S. Brandspigel, M. E. Betz, D. K. Novins, and R. Agans. 2018. Hospital emergency department lethal means counseling for suicidal patients. *American Journal of Preventive Medicine* 54(2):259–265.

RWJF (Robert Wood Johnson Foundation). 2011. *Health care's blind side: The overlooked connection between social needs and good health.* Princeton, NJ: Robert Wood Johnson Foundation.

SAMHSA (Substance Abuse and Mental Health Services Administration). 2014. *SAMHSA's concept of trauma and guidance for a trauma-informed approach.* Rockville, MD: Substance Abuse and Mental Health Services Administration.

Shelton, R. C., D. A. Chambers, and R. E. Glasgow. 2020. An extension of RE-AIM to enhance sustainability: Addressing dynamic context and promoting health equity over time. *Frontiers in Public Health* 8:134. doi:10.3389/fpubh.2020.00134.

Shelton, R. C., P. Adsul, A. Oh, N. Moise, and D. M. Griffith. 2021. Application of an antiracism lens in the field of implementation science (IS): Recommendations for reframing implementation research with a focus on justice and racial equity. *Implementation Research and Practice* 2. https://doi.org/10.1177/26334895211049482 (accessed August 30, 2022).

Shonkoff, J. P., and A. S. Garner. 2012. The lifelong effects of early childhood adversity and toxic stress. *Pediatrics* 129(1):e232–e246.

Siry, B. J., C. E. Knoepke, S. M. Ernestus, D. D. Matlock, and M. E. Betz. 2021a. Lethal means counseling for suicidal adults in the emergency department: A qualitative study. *Western Journal of Emergency Medicine* 22(3):471–477.

Siry, B. J., E. Polzer, F. Omeragic, C. E. Knoepke, D. D. Matlock, and M. E. Betz. 2021b. Lethal means counseling for suicide prevention: Views of emergency department clinicians. *General Hospital Psychiatry* 71:95–101.

Spitzer, S. A., K. L. Staudenmayer, L. Tennakoon, D. A. Spain, and T. G. Weiser. 2017. Costs and financial burden of initial hospitalizations for firearm injuries in the United States, 2006-2014. *American Journal of Public Health* 107(5):770–774. https://doi.org/10.2105/ajph.2017.303684.

Stevens, C. D., D. L. Schriger, B. Raffetto, A. C. Davis, D. Zingmond, and D. H. Roby. 2014. Geographic clustering of diabetic lower-extremity amputations in low-income regions of California. *Health Affairs* 33(8):1383–1390. https://doi.org/10.1377/hlthaff.2014.0148.

The King Center. n.d. *The King philosophy-noviolence365.* https://thekingcenter.org/about-tkc/the-king-philosophy/ (accessed August 10, 2022).

UChicago Medicine. 2021. *At the forefront of health equity 2021 community benefit report.* https://www.uchicagomedicine.org/-/media/pdfs/adult-pdfs/community/community%20benefit%20report/community-benefit-report-brochure-2021 (accessed August 11, 2022).

VA (U.S. Department of Veterans Affairs). 2021. *National veteran suicide prevention annual report.* https://www.mentalhealth.va.gov/docs/data-sheets/2021/2021-National-Veteran-Suicide-Prevention-Annual-Report-FINAL-9-8-21.pdf (accessed August 11, 2022).

Wezerek, G. 2014. *How the L.A. Times is honoring homicide victims through data visualization.* https://www.fastcompany.com/3025582/map-of-la-homicides-honors-the-dead-with-skilled-reporting (accessed August 10, 2022).

Wintemute, G. J., A. J. Aubel, R. Pallin, J. P. Schleimer, and N. Kravitz-Wirtz. 2022. Experiences of violence in daily life among adults in California: A population-representative survey. *Injury Epidemiology* 9(1):1.

Youth Alive! n.d. *Caught in the crossfire.* https://www.youthalive.org/results/ (accessed June 30, 2022).

B

Workshop Agenda

Facilitating the Integration of Firearm Injury Prevention into Health Care Through Community Collaboration: A Workshop

April 25, 2022 | 12:00–5:15 p.m. ET

12:00–12:20 p.m. Opening Remarks

                      Victor Dzau, M.D.
                      President, National Academy of Medicine

                      Michael Dowling, M.D.
                      President and CEO of Northwell Health

                      Jose Prince, M.D.
                      Professor of Surgery and Pediatrics, Zucker School of Medicine at Hofstra/Northwell; Vice Chair of Surgery, Surgeon-in-Chief at Cohen Children's Medical Center; Vice President and Chief of Pediatric Surgery and Acute Care Surgery at Northwell Health

                      Bernard Rosof, M.D.
                      Cochair, Project M.D.
                      PEACE Initiative

12:20–12:35 p.m.   Introductory Session
Framing of the Issue: Firearm Injuries and Health Care's Role in Depolarizing a Public Health Crisis

>Moderator: Megan L. Ranney, M.D., M.P.H.
Academic Dean, School of Public Health, Brown University; Director, Brown-Lifespan Center for Digital Health; and Endowed Professor of Emergency Medicine, Warren Alpert Medical School

>Debra Houry, M.D., M.P.H.
Acting Principal Deputy Director of CDC and Director of the National Center for Injury Prevention and Control (NCIPC) at CDC

12:35–1:35 p.m.   Panel 1:
Health Care Strategies to Reduce Firearm Injury and Mortality

>Moderator: Frederick Rivara, M.D., M.P.H.
Seattle Children's Guild Association Endowed Chair in Pediatrics; Vice Chair and Professor of Pediatrics; Adjunct Professor of Epidemiology, University of Washington; Editor-in-Chief of *JAMA Network Open*

>Thea James, M.D.
Associate Professor of Emergency Medicine, Boston Medical Center/Boston University School of Medicine; Director of the Boston Medical Center site of the Massachusetts Violence Intervention Advocacy Program (VIAP)

>Rochelle Dicker, M.D.
Professor of Surgery and Anesthesia and Vice Chair for Critical Care, Trauma Medical Director, Codirector of the Program for the Advancement of Surgical Equity, UCLA

APPENDIX B   *75*

                    Amy Barnhorst, M.D.
                    Director, BulletPoints Project, California Firearm Violence Research Center; Vice Chair for Clinical Services, Department of Psychiatry and Behavioral Sciences, Associate Clinical Professor, Department of Emergency Medicine, University of California, Davis

                    Discussion

1:35–1:45 p.m.   10 minute break

1:45–2:50 p.m.   Panel 2:
                    Barriers and Facilitators to Implementing Hospital-Based Firearm Injury Prevention Strategies in Urban and Rural Communities

                    Moderator: Andre Campbell, M.D.
                    Professor and Vice Chair of the Department of Surgery, UCSF School of Medicine; Attending Trauma Surgeon, Zuckerberg San Francisco General Hospital and Trauma Center

                    Rinad Beidas, Ph.D.
                    Founder and Director of the Penn Implementation Science Center at the Leonard Davis Institute (PISCE@LDI) and Associate Director at the Center for Health Incentives and Behavioral Economics, University of Pennsylvania

                    Ashley Hink, M.D., M.P.H.
                    Assistant Professor, Acute Care Surgery, Medical University of South Carolina Medical Director, MUSC Turning the Tide Violence Intervention Program (TTVIP)

                    Scott Charles, M.A.P.P.
                    Trauma Outreach Manager, Temple University Hospital and Director of Temple University Hospital's Cradle to Grave Program

                    LeVon Stone, Sr., M.A.
                    CEO and Cofounder of Acclivus, Inc.

                    Sheila Regan
                    Chief Operating Officer of Acclivus, Inc.

                    Discussion

2:50–3:40 p.m.   Panel 3:
                    Collaborating with Communities to Improve Health Care System Implementation Success and Destigmatize Gun Violence Prevention

                    Moderator: Marian (Emmy) Betz, M.D., M.P.H.
                    Professor of Emergency Medicine, Director of the Firearm Injury Prevention Initiative, University of Colorado School of Medicine; Research Physician at the Geriatric Research, Education, and Clinical Core

                    LJ Punch, M.D.
                    Executive Director and founder of The T, St. Louis; Medical Director and Founder of the BRIC (Bullet Related Injury Clinic)

                    Jake Wiskerchen, M.A.
                    Founder, Chief Executive Officer of Zephyr Wellness

                    Rev. Michael McBride
                    Executive Director of LiveFree USA

                    Discussion

3:40–3:50 p.m.   10 minute break

APPENDIX B 77

3:50–4:50 p.m.   Panel 4:
Defining a Firearms Violence Prevention Road Map for Hospitals and Health Systems

Moderator: Chethan Sathya, M.D. M.Sc.
Director of Northwell Health Gun Violence Prevention Center, Pediatric General and Thoracic Surgeon; Associate Medical Director of Trauma, Surgical Director of Pediatric Critical Care at Cohen Children's Medical Center, Northwell Health; Assistant Professor, Zucker School of Medicine at Hofstra/Northwell

James Braxton
Violence Reduction Administrative Coordinator, National Institute for Criminal Justice Reform

Megan L. Ranney, M.D., M.P.H.
Academic Dean, School of Public Health, Brown University; Director, Brown-Lifespan Center for Digital Health; and Endowed Professor of Emergency Medicine, Warren Alpert Medical School

Tom Jackiewicz, M.P.H.
President of University of Chicago Medical Center

Rajeev Ramchand, Ph.D.
Codirector, RAND Epstein Family Veterans Policy Research Institute; senior behavioral scientist, RAND Corporation

Discussion

4:50–5:15 p.m.   Closing Remarks

Joseph Sakran, M.D., M.P.H, M.P.A.
Director of Emergency General Surgery, Associate Professor of Surgery and Nursing, Vice Chair of Clinical Operations, Johns Hopkins Hospital

C

Statement of Task

An ad hoc planning committee of the National Academies of Sciences, Engineering, and Medicine will host a 1-day public workshop to be conducted jointly with Northwell Health and PEACE Initiative. The workshop will bring together firearm injury prevention thought leaders to explore how hospitals, health systems, and the health care industry at large can integrate interventions for firearm injury prevention into routine care for the purpose of improving the health and safety of patients and communities.

The workshop will explore a broad range of topics including:

- The state of evidence on health care strategies to reduce firearm injury and mortality
- Barriers to implementing health care strategies:
  - Patient/survivor perceptions and barriers to discussing firearm injury prevention with clinical team members
  - Provider perspectives
- Factors that facilitate the implementation of health care strategies
- How to adapt and implement public health and harm-reduction strategies across a variety of health care settings (emergency departments, surgery, primary care settings)
- The need for diverse perspectives in shaping health care firearm injury harm-reduction strategies:
  - Patient/survivors
  - Owners of firearms
  - Community-based voices (community-based organizations)

- Key elements of a health care industry road map for overcoming barriers to integrating harm-reduction and public health strategies around firearm injury prevention into routine care

A planning committee will plan and organize the workshop, select and invite speakers and discussants, and moderate the discussions. A proceedings of the presentations and discussions at the workshop will be prepared by a designated *rapporteur* in accordance with institutional guidelines. The proceedings will be subject to an appropriate review procedure prior to release.

D

Biographical Sketches of the Speakers and Moderators

Amy Barnhorst, M.D., *Director, BulletPoints Project, California Firearm Violence Research Center; Vice Chair for Clinical Services, Department of Psychiatry and Behavioral Sciences, Associate Clinical Professor, Department of Emergency Medicine, University of California, Davis*
Amy Barnhorst, M.D., is an emergency and inpatient psychiatrist whose work doing violence and suicide risk assessments led to her interest in firearm injury prevention. She is a nationally recognized expert on firearms laws and mental illness, and her academic work focuses on the interface between firearms, violence, suicide, and mental illness. Drawing on her previous experience as an outdoor educator, she is active in medical education, and works with both state and federal legislators to craft evidence-based firearm laws. She has presented nationally on these topics, and has written about them for the *New York Times* and *Slate*. Currently, she is leading the BulletPoints Project, funded by the State of California, to develop and disseminate a firearm injury prevention curriculum to health care providers. Dr. Barnhorst became involved in gun violence prevention after the Sandy Hook shooting. After joining the Consortium for Risk-Based Firearm Policy in 2014, she helped contribute to the development and implementation of California's Gun Violence Restraining Order. With other consortium researchers, she has presented on expert panels in multiple states to help educate legislators about the evidence behind various firearm-related policies. She has written multiple academic papers on firearms, mental illness, and the law and was featured in the *New York Times*, the *Sacramento Bee*, and on her blog at *Psychology Today*.

Rinad Beidas, Ph.D., *Founder and Director of the Penn Implementation Science Center at the Leonard Davis Institute (PISCE@LDI), Director of the Penn Medicine Nudge Unit, University of Pennsylvania*
Rinad Beidas, Ph.D., is the Director of the Penn Medicine Nudge Unit; Founder and Director of the Penn Implementation Science Center at the Leonard Davis Institute (PISCE@LDI); and Associate Director at the Center for Health Incentives and Behavioral Economics (CHIBE). She is a Professor of Medical Ethics and Health Policy and Psychiatry at the University of Pennsylvania. Her research program is designed to improve the quality of health care delivery through implementation science. One foci of her research includes implementing evidence-based firearm safety promotion approaches in pediatric primary care settings as a universal suicide prevention strategy. She partners with a diverse set of stakeholders, including gun owner constituents, to understand how best to realize this goal.

Moderator: Marian (Emmy) Betz, M.D., M.P.H., *Professor of Emergency Medicine, Director of the Firearm Injury Prevention Initiative, University of Colorado School of Medicine; Research Physician at the Geriatric Research, Education, and Clinical Core, Eastern Colorado VA*
Emmy Betz, M.D., M.P.H., is a board-certified emergency physician who works clinically at the University of Colorado Hospital and leads a large research program in firearm injury prevention. She is currently a Professor of Emergency Medicine at the University of Colorado School of Medicine, Director of the Firearm Injury Prevention Initiative at the Injury and Violence Prevention Center at the University of Colorado Anschutz Medical Campus, and a Research Physician at the Geriatric Research, Education, and Clinical Core for the Eastern Colorado VA. She is a nationally recognized expert in firearm injury prevention and suicide prevention and has served as a subject-matter expert with numerous medical organizations and the Department of Defense Suicide Prevention Office. She cofounded and leads the Colorado Firearm Safety Coalition, a collaborative effort between public health and medical professionals and firearm retailers to reduce firearm suicides. She serves as principal investigator and coinvestigator on multiple research projects funded through the National Institutes of Health and private foundations, she has published more than 130 peer-reviewed manuscripts, and in 2015 she gave a TEDxMileHigh talk on firearm suicide.

James Braxton, *Violence Reduction Administrative Coordinator, National Institute for Criminal Justice Reform*
Newport News, Virginia, native James E. Braxton II, is a father of two and founder of SoulStrong Outreach & Consulting LLC. Mr. Braxton's lived experience and continued fight for youth justice, violence prevention, and

strengthening families enables him to encourage affected families to exceed their goals in the face of extreme adversity. He is nationally known as the "Transformation Expert" and "Master Career Coach," with a diverse skill set to match his desire to see people grow beyond boundaries. In 2016, he was selected to deliver the commencement speech for the graduating class of Thomas Jefferson High School in Richmond, Virginia. Mr. Braxton's trauma-informed approach to youth development and community outreach led him to publish his first children's book in 2020 titled *SoulStrong: Heroes of Trauma*. He currently serves as the Violence Reduction Administrative Coordinator for the National Institute for Criminal Justice Reform, where he continues his fight for youth justice and systems transformation.

Andre Campbell, M.D., *Professor and Vice Chair of the Department of Surgery, University of California, San Francisco School of Medicine; Attending Trauma Surgeon, Zuckerberg San Francisco General Hospital and Trauma Center*
Andre Campbell, M.D., FACS, FACP, FCCM, MAMSE, FCCOS, is the Professor and Vice Chair of the Department of Surgery, University of California, San Francisco School of Medicine. He is an attending trauma surgeon at the Zuckerberg San Francisco General Hospital. Dr. Campbell has cared for gunshot wound victims for three decades in inner city hospitals in New York and San Francisco. He is an award-winning educator, master surgeon, researcher, and health care leader and has been an advocate for victims of violent crime for his entire career. He has mentored an entire generation of physician and surgeons during his long career. He has won multiple awards for his service to his community.

Scott Charles, M.A.P.P., *Trauma Outreach Manager and Director of the Cradle to Grave Program, Temple University Hospital*
Scott Charles , M.A.P.P., is the Trauma Outreach Manager for Temple University Hospital and is Director of the hospital's Cradle to Grave program, an award-winning, hospital-based violence prevention initiative that educates public school students and adjudicated youth about the medical realities of firearm injury. He also coordinates the hospital's Trauma Victims Support Advocates program that connects violently injured patients to crime victim services throughout Philadelphia. Mr. Charles also directs the hospital's Fighting Chance program, which teaches community members to provide first aid to victims of gunshot injury, as well as the Safe Bet program, which has distributed more than 8,000 free gun locks to city residents. His work with trauma surgeon Dr. Amy Goldberg has been showcased on CNN, CBS News, ABC World News, MSNBC, Huffington Post, and NPR's Fresh Air with Terry Gross. Their work has also been featured in the *New York Times* and in the HBO documentary "Gun Fight." Mr. Charles holds degrees in psychology from the University of Pennsylvania.

Rochelle Dicker, M.D., *Professor of Surgery and Anesthesia and Vice Chair for Critical Care, University of California, Los Angeles; Codirector, Program for the Advancement of Surgical Equity*
Rochelle Dicker, M.D., is Professor of Surgery at the University of California, Los Angeles (UCLA). She serves as the Vice Chair for Critical Care and the Trauma Medical Director. She also cochairs the UCLA Health Equity and Translational Social Science Theme for the School of Medicine and is codirector of the Program for the Advancement of Surgical Equity. In 2005 she founded the Wraparound Project at San Francisco General Hospital. Wraparound is a hospital-based violence intervention program based on a public health model. Wraparound was one of six start-up programs that formed the National Network of Hospital-Based Violence Intervention Programs. Now called the Health Alliance for Violence Intervention, this organization is home to more than 80 programs. Dr. Dicker is the Advisory Board Chair. She is a member of the American College of Surgeons Committee on Trauma where she leads a group called Improving the Social Determinants to Attenuate Violence. The group works to integrate social care models and trauma-informed practices across the country in trauma centers.

Michael Dowling, M.D., *President and CEO of Northwell Health*
Michael Dowling, M.D., is one of health care's most influential voices, leading a clinical, academic, and research enterprise with a workforce of more than 78,000 and annual revenue of $15 billion. Prior to joining Northwell in 1995, he served in New York State government for 12 years as the chief health and human services advisor to former Governor Mario Cuomo, and was a professor of social policy at Fordham University. He has been a recipient of the Columbia School of Business' Deming Cup, the Ellis Island Medal of Honor, and the Presidential Distinguished Service Award for Irish Abroad, and he served as the 2017 Grand Marshal of the St. Patrick's Day parade in New York City.

Victor J. Dzau, M.D., *President, National Academy of Medicine*
Victor J. Dzau, M.D., is the President of the National Academy of Medicine (NAM), formerly the Institute of Medicine (IOM). In addition, he serves as Chair of the IOM Division Committee of the National Academies of Sciences, Engineering, and Medicine. Dr. Dzau has made a significant impact on medicine through his seminal research in cardiovascular medicine and genetics, pioneering the discipline of vascular medicine, and leadership in health care innovation. In his role as a leader in health care, Dr. Dzau has led efforts in health care innovation. His vision is for academic health sciences centers to lead the transformation of medicine through innovation, translation, and globalization. In addition to his work with the IOM, Dr. Dzau is currently a

member of the Board of Directors of the Singapore Health System, Governing Board of Duke-National University of Singapore Graduate Medical School, and Senior Health Policy Advisor to Her Highness Sheikha Moza (Chair of the Qatar Foundation). He is also on the Board of Health Governors of the World Economic Forum and chaired its Global Agenda Council on Personalized and Precision Medicine. He is Chancellor Emeritus for Health Affairs and James B. Duke Professor of Medicine at Duke University and the past President and CEO of the Duke University Health System. Previously, Dr. Dzau was the Hersey Professor of Theory and Practice of Medicine and Chairman of Medicine at Harvard Medical School's Brigham and Women's Hospital, as well as Chairman of the Department of Medicine at Stanford University.

Ashley Hink, M.D., M.P.H., *Assistant Professor of Acute Care Surgery, Medical Director, MUSC Turning the Tide Violence Intervention Program, Medical University of South Carolina*
Ashley Hink, M.D., M.P.H., is a trauma, burn, and critical care surgeon in Charleston, South Carolina, at the Medical University of South Carolina (MUSC). In addition to her clinical interests and surgical practice, she is a public health researcher focusing on risk factors for violent injuries, health care strategies to support victims of violence, and recovery after injury. She serves on the American College of Surgeons Committee on Trauma Injury Prevention and Control Committee, working on research and advocacy efforts to address violence as a public health problem. She is the Founder and Medical Director of the first hospital-based violence intervention program in South Carolina, the MUSC Turning the Tide Violence Intervention Program and has received funding from the National Collaborative on Gun Violence Research and the U.S. Department of Justice for research and program implementation.

Debra Houry, M.D., M.P.H., *Acting Principal Deputy Director, Centers for Disease Control and Prevention*
Since 2014, Debra Houry, M.D., M.P.H., has served as Director of the National Center for Injury Prevention and Control at the Centers for Disease Control and Prevention. Dr. Houry previously served as an associate professor at Emory University and emergency physician at Grady Memorial Hospital. Dr. Houry received her M.D. and M.P.H. degrees from Tulane University and completed her residency training in emergency medicine at Denver Health Medical Center.

Tom Jackiewicz, M.P.H., *President of University of Chicago Medicine*
Tom Jackiewicz, M.P.H., is President of UChicago Medicine, the $2.5 billion academic and community health system that includes the University of Chicago Medical Center, the Biological Sciences Division, the Pritzker School

of Medicine, and UChicago Medicine Ingalls Memorial. Mr. Jackiewicz leads the clinical enterprise, including the integration of the patient care mission of the medical center with the education and research missions of the University of Chicago Biological Sciences Division. His career has focused on executing ambitious and broad transformation in academic environments and engaging physician leaders to drive organizational change. A strategic visionary, he has ushered in eras of substantial growth and improvement at academic health systems across the country, including Keck Medicine of the University of Southern California, University of California, San Diego Health System and School of Medicine, Columbia University Medical Center, and Stanford School of Medicine.

Thea James, M.D., *Associate Professor of Emergency Medicine, Boston Medical Center/Boston University School of Medicine; Director of the Boston Medical Center site of the Massachusetts Violence Intervention Advocacy Program (VIAP)*
Thea James, M.D., is an Associate Professor of Emergency Medicine at Boston Medical Center/Boston University School of Medicine, President of the Boston Medical and Dental Staff, Vice President of Mission, and Associate Chief Medical Officer. She is also the Director of the Boston Medical Center site of the Massachusetts Violence Intervention Advocacy Program (VIAP). Boston Medical Center's VIAP program helps guide victims of community violence through recovery from physical and emotional trauma. Her diversity areas of interest include African American culture, LGBT, and women in medicine. Dr. James has chaired and served on national committees within the Society for Academic Emergency Medicine (SAEM), served as a moderator, and has given public lectures and talks. She was appointed to the SAEM Women in Academic Emergency Medicine Task Force, is a member of the Boston University School of Medicine Admissions Committee, and in 2009, was appointed to the Massachusetts Board of Registration in Medicine, where she presently serves as chair of the Licensing Committee. Dr. James is the 2008 awardee of the Mulligan Award for public service.

Rev. Michael McBride, *Executive Director of LiveFree USA*
Pastor Michael McBride is a native of San Francisco and has been active in ministry for more than 20 years. He is the Executive Director of LIVE FREE USA, a nonprofit committed to ending gun violence, mass incarceration, and the death penalty. Regarded as a national faith leader, Pastor McBride was active in the Ferguson uprisings and subsequent protest movements. He helps bridge, train, and support millennials and religious institutions working on racial justice and Black liberation. He has served on a number of local and national task forces with the White House and Department of Justice regarding gun violence prevention, boys and men of color, and police–community relationships.

Jose M. Prince, M.D., *Professor, Surgery and Pediatrics, Donald and Barbara Zucker School of Medicine at Hofstra/Northwell*
Jose M. Prince, M.D., FACS, FAAP, is a Professor of Surgery and Pediatrics at the Zucker School of Medicine at Hofstra/Northwell, Vice Chair of Surgery, the Surgeon-in-Chief at Cohen Children's Medical Center, and Northwell Health's Vice President and Chief of Pediatric Surgery and Acute Care Surgery. He is also the Founding Director of the Laboratory of Pediatric Injury and Inflammation at the Feinstein Institutes for Medical Research. A nationally recognized expert in pediatric trauma, he is a member of the Committee on Trauma of the American College of Surgeons and a leader in teaching minimally invasive neonatal surgery. He has been invited to speak internationally about his research, teaching, and clinical activities. He has authored more than 60 articles in peer-reviewed journals, in addition to numerous clinical and scientific chapters.

LJ Punch, M.D., *Executive Director and founder of "The T" and Medical Director and founder of the BRIC*
LJ Punch, M.D., is a transmasculine, nonbinary, biracial, neurodiverse human who loves to heal. Educated in medicine at the University of Connecticut and trained in surgery at the University of Maryland and Shock Trauma Center in Baltimore, this desire to heal has brought to life a career with a three-fold focus: education, trauma, and equity. Moving to Ferguson post-Ferguson to be on the faculty at Washington University in St. Louis School of Medicine, this work came to life for him in the development of a wide variety of educational and clinical resources in the management of surgical emergencies across the entire spectrum of illness and healing. In 2018 he collaborated with numerous health care professionals, students, and community members to create "The T," a community of health working to reduce the impact of trauma through broad public health campaigns, mobile outreach, and brick-and-mortar services. In the wake of the pandemic, he left academic medicine to be the Executive Director of The T with an expanded focus on multiple sources of trauma disproportionately experienced by Black people including COVID-19, bullet injuries, and opioid dependence. This includes the creation of the Bullet Related Injury Clinic, or the BRIC, a community-based free clinic for patients and their loved ones who are discharged from the emergency department after being shot, with a focus on the experience of the Black masculine body.

Rajeev Ramchand, Ph.D., *Codirector of the RAND Epstein Family Veterans Policy Research Institute and senior behavioral scientist, RAND Corporation*
Rajeev Ramchand, Ph.D., is Codirector of the RAND Epstein Family Veterans Policy Research Institute and a senior behavioral scientist at the RAND

Corporation. He studies the prevalence, prevention, and treatment of mental health and substance use disorders in adolescents, service members and veterans, and minority populations. He has conducted many studies on suicide and suicide prevention including environmental scans of suicide prevention programs, epidemiologic studies on risk factors for suicide, qualitative research with suicide loss survivors, and evaluations of suicide prevention programs. He has also developed freely available tools to help organizations evaluate their own suicide prevention programs. He has testified on suicide prevention before the United States Senate, House of Representatives, and California State Senate. Other current areas of research include military and veteran caregivers; the role of firearm availability, storage, and policies on suicide; the impact of disasters on community health; and using public health approaches to study and prevent hate and violent extremism.

Megan L. Ranney, M.D., M.P.H., FACEP, *Academic Dean, School of Public Health; Director, Brown-Lifespan Center for Digital Health; Warren Alpert Endowed Professor of Emergency Medicine*
Megan L. Ranney, M.D., M.P.H., FACEP, is a practicing emergency physician, researcher, and national advocate for innovative approaches to public health. She is the Academic Dean at the School of Public Health at Brown University, the Warren Alpert Endowed Professor of Emergency Medicine at Alpert Medical School of Brown University, and Founding Director of the Brown-Lifespan Center for Digital Health. Dr. Ranney's research focuses on developing, testing, and disseminating digital health interventions to prevent violence and related behavioral health problems, as well as on COVID-related risk reduction. She has received numerous awards for technology innovation, public health, and research, including Rhode Island Woman of the Year and the American College of Emergency Physicians' Policy Pioneer Award. She is also a frequent media commentator on outlets ranging from the BBC to CNN to the *New York Times*.

Sheila Regan, *Chief Operating Officer of Acclivus, Inc.*
Sheila Regan has worked in multiple roles on research projects in this realm including study design, development, data systems development, abstract/manuscript writing, and data analysis. Ms. Regan has played an integral role in the development of the Cure Violence Illinois hospital intervention, starting as an external partner employed by Mount Sinai Hospital, a local level 1 trauma center. As the hospital program director from 2007 to 2013, Ms. Regan was solely responsible for oversight of 24/7 operations of the program in Chicago, development of program structure and foundational documents as well as technical assistance to Cure Violence replication sites nationally. Prior to her time with Cure Violence, she worked directly with violently injured

patients, including injury by sexual, domestic, shooting, stabbing, and other violence, as the Crime Victim Advocate for Mount Sinai Hospital. Since 2000, she has worked as an advocate for individuals experiencing sexual abuse and/or domestic violence and has certification working with both populations. She completed her bachelor of science at the University of Illinois Urbana-Champaign in 2004 and was a recipient of the National Merit Scholarship in 2000.

Frederick P. Rivara, M.D., M.P.H., *Seattle Children's Guild Association Endowed Chair in Pediatrics, Vice Chair and Professor of Pediatrics, Adjunct Professor of Epidemiology, University of Washington; Editor-in-Chief of* JAMA Network Open
Frederick P. Rivara, M.D., M.P.H., is the holder of the Seattle Children's Guild Association Endowed Chair in Pediatrics, and he is Vice Chair and Professor of Pediatrics and adjunct Professor of Epidemiology at the University of Washington (UW). He is editor-in-chief of *JAMA Network Open*. He served as Founding Director of the Harborview Injury and Research Center in Seattle for 13 years and has devoted his career to studying injury and injury prevention. He has received numerous honors including the Charles C. Shepard Science Award from the Centers for Disease Control and Prevention, the American Public Health Association, Injury Control and Emergency Health Services Section Distinguished Career Award, the American Academy of Pediatrics, Section on Injury and Poison Prevention, Physician Achievement Award, the UW School of Public Health Distinguished Alumni Award, and the UW Medicine Minority Faculty Mentoring Award. Dr. Rivara was elected to the Institute of Medicine (now National Academy of Medicine) in 2005. He was awarded the Joseph St. Geme, Jr., Leadership Award from the Federation of Pediatric Organizations in 2021. He has conducted firearms-related research since 1987 and currently directs the Firearm Injury and Policy Research Program in the Harborview Injury Prevention and Research Center at the University of Washington.

Bernard Rosof, M.D., *PEACE Initiative*
Bernard Rosof, M.D., is a clinical gastroenterologist having practiced internal medicine and gastroenterology for 29 years. He is on the Board of Directors of Huntington Hospital (Northwell Health System) and is the past chair, and he is on the Board of Advisors of the Northwell Health System. He is Professor of Medicine at the Zucker School of Medicine at Hofstra/Northwell. Dr. Rosof is Board Chairman of the Institute for Exceptional Care. He has chaired many committees for the National Academies of Sciences, Engineering, and Medicine; specialty societies; and national and state initiatives in quality and performance improvement.

Joseph V. Sakran, M.D., M.P.H., M.P.A., FACS, *Director of Emergency General Surgery, Associate Professor of Surgery and Nursing, Vice Chair of Clinical Operations, John Hopkins Hospital*
Joseph V. Sakran, M.D., M.P.H., M.P.A., FACS, is a trauma surgeon, coalition builder, policy advisor, public health practitioner, and nationally recognized advocate for gun violence prevention. He is currently Director of Emergency General Surgery, Associate Professor of Surgery and Nursing, and Vice Chair of Clinical Operations at the Johns Hopkins Hospital in Baltimore, Maryland. Dr. Sakran is also a Senior Fellow at the Satcher Health Leadership Institute at the Morehouse School of Medicine. A survivor of gun violence himself, Dr. Sakran's interest in medicine and trauma surgery began after a stray bullet nearly killed him during his senior year of high school. He has subsequently dedicated his life to treating the most vulnerable, reducing health disparities among marginalized populations, and advancing public policy that alleviates structural violence in low-income communities.

Dr. Chethan Sathya, M.D., M.Sc., *Director of Northwell Health Gun Violence Prevention Center, Pediatric General and Thoracic Surgeon; Associate Medical Director of Trauma, Surgical Director of Pediatric Critical Care at Cohen Children's Medical Center, Northwell Health; Assistant Professor, Zucker School of Medicine at Hofstra/Northwell*
Dr. Chethan Sathya, M.D., M.Sc., is a pediatric trauma surgeon and National Institutes of Health (NIH)-funded firearm injury prevention researcher. He serves as Director of Northwell Health's Center for Gun Violence Prevention and oversees the health system's expansive approach to firearm injury prevention. Northwell Health, the largest health system in New York State, has taken a public health approach to gun violence prevention, focusing on key areas such as research, medical education, clinical screening, advocacy, and community engagement. Dr. Sathya was recently awarded $1.4 million from the NIH to study gun violence prevention and implement a first-of-its-kind protocol to universally screen those at risk of firearm injury. The grant is part of the health system's "We Ask Everyone. Firearm Safety is a Health Issue" research study, which aims to shift the paradigm to view gun violence as a public health issue and approach firearm injury risk similarly to other health risk factors like smoking and substance use. Furthermore, Dr. Sathya spearheaded the formation of the National Gun Violence Prevention Learning Collaborative for Hospitals and Health Systems, in which hospitals can learn about gun violence prevention from experts, develop best practices, and implement strategies to prevent firearm injuries. Dr. Sathya is Associate Trauma Director at Cohen Children's Medical Center and Assistant Professor of Surgery and Pediatrics at the Donald and Barbara Zucker School of Medicine at Hofstra/Northwell. He completed medical school and general surgery training at the University of Toronto, followed

by a pediatric surgery fellowship at Northwestern Medicine in Chicago. He also holds a master's in clinical epidemiology from the University of Toronto, in addition to fellowships in global journalism and public health.

LeVon Stone, Sr., M.A., *CEO and Cofounder of Acclivus Inc.*

LeVon Stone, Sr., M.A., is the Chief Executive Officer of Acclivus, Inc., a community health organization focused on employing grassroots leaders from Chicago to support safety, well-being, and growth in vulnerable communities. He has been an example of growth and development for individuals from communities across the social landscape. Mr. Stone serves as the CEO, and in his role, he brings voice to victims of violence, as a leader for people facing what feels like insurmountable trials. Over the course of his professional growth within the field, Mr. Stone returned to school, completing a bachelor's and then a master's degree from Northeastern Illinois University with a focus in inner city studies. In his violence prevention work, he has risen through the ranks of the Cure Violence/CeaseFire program, beginning as a volunteer, then consistently promoted from Violence Interrupter to Hospital Responder to Case Manager to Hospital Program Director, and finally holding the highest title possible, Program Director for the State of Illinois. Mr. Stone has successfully advocated for comprehensive services for those acutely at risk for violence by working closely and transparently with government leaders at city, county, and state levels; philanthropic leaders; health and human service providers; and academic partners. This professional experience managing close to $10 million dollars in funds prepared him well to branch out and develop his own independent, Black-led community organization serving violently injured patients at local trauma centers—Acclivus, Inc.

Jake Wiskerchen, M.A., *Founder, Chief Executive Officer, Zephyr Wellness*

Jake Wiskerchen, M.A., is a marriage and family therapist licensed in Nevada, as well as a National Certified Counselor. He owns Zephyr Wellness, a mental health outpatient practice in northern Nevada and spent 2 years chairing his licensing board where he helped rewrite most of his state's laws that govern the profession. As a Walk the Talk America board member and lifelong gun owner, Mr. Wiskerchen is bringing together the communities of firearms and mental health with the goal of improving psychological well-being and preventing firearm suicide. By offering firearms cultural competence courses for practitioners and classes to demystify counseling to gun owners, he hopes to remove barriers to care access, both actual and perceived.